GOOD ENOUGH

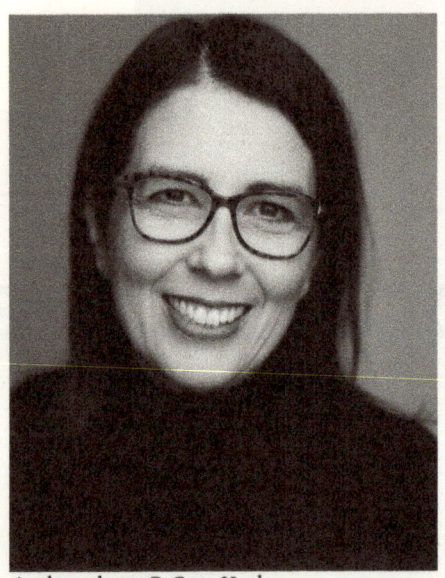

Author photo © Cam Harle

Dr Tara Porter is a clinical psychologist and author. She worked for the NHS for 28 years and now works in private practice. Her specialisms include eating disorders; mental health; education; teenage girls and parenting. She writes and teaches about mental health in the mainstream media and in education settings. She is an associate tutor at UCL. Her first book *You Don't Understand Me: The Young Woman's Guide to Life*, published in 2022, was a *Sunday Times* bestseller and sold in 20 other countries around the world.

GOOD ENOUGH

A Framework for Modern Parents

by

Dr Tara Porter

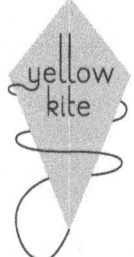

First published in Great Britain in 2025 by Yellow Kite
An imprint of Hodder & Stoughton Limited
An Hachette UK company

The authorised representative in the EEA is Hachette Ireland, 8 Castlecourt Centre, Dublin 15, D15 XTP3, Ireland (email: info@hbgi.ie)

1

Copyright © Dr Tara Porter 2025

The right of Tara Porter to be identified as the Author of the Work has been asserted by her in accordance with the Copyright, Designs and Patents Act 1988.

Epigraph by William Martin, from *The Parent's Tao Te Ching*, copyright © 1999, used with permission, arranged by Barbara Moulton at the Moulton Agency.

Photo on page 32 reproduced with permission of the Harlow Primate Laboratory, University of Wisconsin-Madison.

Quote on page 36 copyright © Katherine May 2018, reproduced with permission of the Licensor through PLSclear.

All rights reserved. No part of this publication may be reproduced, stored in a retrieval system, or transmitted, in any form or by any means without the prior written permission of the publisher, nor be otherwise circulated in any form of binding or cover other than that in which it is published and without a similar condition being imposed on the subsequent purchaser.

A CIP catalogue record for this title is available from the British Library

Hardback ISBN 9781399736077
Trade Paperback ISBN 9781399744232
ebook ISBN 9781399736060

Typeset in Celeste by Manipal Technologies Limited

Printed and bound in Great Britain by Clays Ltd, Elcograf S.p.A.

Hodder & Stoughton policy is to use papers that are natural, renewable and recyclable products and made from wood grown in sustainable forests. The logging and manufacturing processes are expected to conform to the environmental regulations of the country of origin.

Hodder & Stoughton Limited
Carmelite House
50 Victoria Embankment
London EC4Y 0DZ

www.yellowkitebooks.co.uk

For My Three.

Do not ask your children
to strive for extraordinary lives.
Such striving may seem admirable,
but it is a way of foolishness.

'Make the Ordinary Come Alive',
William Martin

CONTENTS

Introduction 1

PART 1: BABIES
1.1 Starting Off Good Enough 17
1.2 Relationship-Based Parenting 30
1.3 Firm and Kind 42
1.4 Your Identity as a Parent 54

PART 2: TODDLERS AND PRE-SCHOOLERS
2.1 Toddler Tantrums, Star Charts and All That Jazz 73
2.2 Play and Joy 92
2.3 Good-Enough Food and Eating 105

PART 3: CHILDHOOD
3.1 The Busyness Business 123
3.2 School and Education 135
3.3 Relationships in Childhood 157
3.4 Screens, the Internet and Phones 178

PART 4: TWEENS AND TEENS

4.1 The Perfect Storm – The Adolescent Years	209
4.2 Holding On and Letting Go	234
4.3 Keeping Your Relationship Going	254
4.4 You, as a Parent with Adolescent and Adult Children	275

Acknowledgements	283
References	285
Index	293

Introduction

'BEING A PARENT MADE ME A WORSE CHILD PSYCHOLOGIST'
I have a very strong memory of observing my supervisor when I was a trainee clinical psychologist on my child placement. I had a chair in the corner of the room, so as to be as inconspicuous as possible. The young parents who had come to see him seemingly didn't notice me, but I think that was partly because they were so desperate for his help. They sat on the edges of their seats, looking at him, my boss, with pleading eyes. They barely paused for breath in their verbal onslaught. A story of eighteen months of broken nights, of screaming and crying, and 'please, tell us what to do'. They were looking at him with the belief that he was *the* guru with the answers.

My supervisor, a man extraordinary only in his ordinariness, did not look like a guru. A sweater-wearing, flat-footed, short man, with a bush of unkempt hair and thick spectacles. But he listened with spectacular intensity and, when they finished, he said, 'Well, there are two truths about this. There is first the truth I would have told before I had a child myself. That truth is that if you want her to stop crying, you need to stop answering her cries. Now, you can do this quickly or gradually; either will work, and there are pros and cons to both. We can talk about those.' He paused, then went on: 'The trouble is that now I am a father I understand just how hard it is to do this. Being a parent has made me a worse child psychologist.'

I didn't have children at the time – it would be another five years until I did – but his words struck a chord in me. I guess as a trainee, I was already beginning to be aware that when I was a psychologist, I would be giving advice, coaching and encouraging people in directions that the non-psychologist me also struggled with. Once I had children, and particularly because the first of my three was a very unsettled baby, my supervisor's words came back to me. As I sat in a rocking chair, delirious with tiredness, trying to soothe my new baby, I thought back to those parents, and all the parents I had seen in the intervening years, and wondered whether I had really understood their experience until then. I feared that I had underestimated how difficult it was. Or worse, that I had patronised them.

From then to now, twenty-four years, every day I have parented with the psychologist me there in the background, too. Sometimes I have used the psychologist part of me wisely in my parenting; I have made parenting decisions in line with my psychological knowledge. At other times, my own emotions have clouded what I believe from research or clinical experience to be true. Sometimes I have hung on to my experience as a psychologist too tightly and it has sent me in the wrong direction as a parent.

But I have also been a psychologist to children and adolescents with my experience as a parent inside me. I have sat with hundreds of children and teenagers, and had to take off my parenting hat to fully understand their perspective. That has looped back into my own understanding of my children.

At times, I have been full of shame, for getting it wrong. Arriving at my NHS job one morning when my children were small, someone gave me an absentminded, cheery morning 'How are you?'

as we stood side by side at the pigeonholes checking our messages. I couldn't bear to be asked. I put my forehead against the pigeonholes and wailed, 'How can I be a child psychologist today, when I've been such an awful mum this morning?' The receptionist glanced over her shoulder and quickly shut the window separating us from the waiting room – not a good look, the psychologist having a breakdown. I don't remember what had happened that morning with my three kids, but I'm pretty sure shouting was involved. Could I be a decent psychologist on mornings like this? Was I a bad parent for not following the advice I doled out to other parents?

From the shame of moments like that, I had to think about my own limitations and failures. I learnt stuff, I grew in both roles and this book is about what I learnt. Firstly, from psychological research and theory; secondly, from my clinical practice over thirty years with children and adolescents; and thirdly, from parenting three children – two boys and a girl – and from my observations of the parents and kids I've known in my personal life over that time.

As a clinical psychologist, I was trained to be a scientific practitioner – to look to the science to guide my clinical practice. But as a parent, there is seemingly no scientific or clinical consensus and on a daily basis there are different experts proposing different theories, or research being summarised into headlines with opposing viewpoints. This is true of many of the topics I discuss in this book, most notably, sleep, toddler behaviour management and screens. In my parenting, my clinical work and, again, writing this book, I have read a tonne of research in its original form. When I do this, I often find points of consensus that are missed in the headlines or expert positions. I have also frequently found a low level of applicability between the research and real family life: there are just too many variables that scientists can't control. On sleep training, for example, what does Granny do if she puts the baby to bed? On temper tantrums, what happens if two children kick off at the same time? Or on phone use, who can really control or measure what an adolescent does on screens? Are we monitoring when they use their friend's phone? Their mum's computer? Their secret IG account? It is partially in this variability that researchers find conflicting results.

I've looked at the differences in the research results and tried to understand them in terms of the design of the many studies – the number of participants, their similarity to real life – and in this book I am drawing my own conclusions. I make no apology for using personal and clinical experience to illustrate points: I am not saying 'this happened to me and so it is true'; what I am saying is that I read this research, I saw these patients clinically and I raised these kids and, putting it all together, this is what I learnt.

UPSTREAM
Client to me: *I don't want to be one of those people who thinks about their parents all the time in therapy. I want to have sorted my own stuff.*
Me to client: *Perhaps you also don't want to be one of those people who rely on oxygen?*

Our parents are a key influence on who we are and who we become as adults. And this is a book about the whole kaleidoscope of that parenting influence. It is a book about babies, toddlers, school-age children, teenagers and young adults; it's about raising a child to be a fully functioning adult.

Why? Mostly in my clinical practice these days I see adolescents and young adults, thirteen- to twenty-five-year-olds, and/or their parents. Often, they are unhappy, anxious and lost in life.

Many of them have diagnoses like OCD, school refusal, anorexia or depression, and they are coming to therapy to be cured. Yet despite this, it can be hard for them to get better; they are already stuck in patterns, and they think they can't change them. Their parents are desperate to help, but often, so often, they wish to turn back time. They can see how the roots of their child's unhappiness were planted earlier.

As a therapist, therefore, I often feel I am trying to undo habitual brain patterns that were set down earlier in life. I'm not a neurologist but, as I understand it, when we get lots of the same message – whether from other people or ourselves – or we repeat a behaviour many times, we end up strengthening certain brain connections in our minds. When these messages or behaviours get extreme, and, of course, depending on someone's genetic loading, the brain can get sucked into mental illness.

Changing habitual thought patterns in therapy is hard work. I enjoy working with young people as they are still developing and changing anyway – their brains are still 'wiring' – whereas older people are more stuck in their ways. But, even so, change in therapy is not easy: it is often torturous and time-consuming. What's more, it's expensive, not widely available and teenagers are suffering when they are anxious and depressed. My point is: the answer to the current mental-health crisis amongst teenagers and young people is not just trying to cure, but also trying to prevent. As is captured in this quote, usually ascribed to South African bishop and theologian Desmond Tutu, 'There comes a point where we need to stop just pulling people out of the river. We need to go upstream and find out why they're falling in.'

MY MANIFESTO FOR MENTAL HEALTH

This is a book about the upstream, about how we parent babies, toddlers, primary-age kids, tweens and teenagers, to reduce the chances that they need to be pulled out of the river downstream. And reflecting on the many adolescents I've seen in my clinical work, I think there are six things we should be aiming for, which, for me, define good mental health. I call these my manifesto for mental health.

Good enough

We, as parents, clinicians and society, get caught up in diagnoses, but when I see mentally unwell teenagers, whatever their diagnosis, nearly all of them don't feel good enough. They feel full of shame at their own being. They don't think they are clever, funny, pretty, nice, popular enough, whatever their actual level of functioning. Not feeling good enough is a cause and a result of mental illness. There is a bit of a gender split on how this feeling expresses itself, as in girls it tends to get internalised, and they do things that hurt themselves, including worrying too much or stopping eating, whereas boys more often externalise the feeling in arrogance and/or violence.

Feeling 'good enough' is less about the frequently cited self-esteem, and more about self-acceptance. So this is my first manifesto aim: I don't want your child necessarily to think they are brilliant, but I definitely don't want them to think everything about them is wrong. I want them to feel good and enough. And through this book, we will be thinking about how you can foster this good-enough feeling upstream, when they are younger.

Balanced anxiety

Your child will inevitably have negative emotions as they grow up. You cannot protect them from this, and nor, indeed, should you want to. Difficult feelings are the shadow to the light – an inevitable and necessary side effect of connection and love. Without them, children would not have full lives; they would be like some sort of precious doll in a box. And so some degree of apprehension and worry are normal in the living of a full, real life.

But I see so many adolescents and young adults with crippling anxiety. Usually, they are trying to control or avoid their anxiety in ways that are hugely unhelpful. They try to control it with unhelpful strategies like starving themselves or developing obsessive rules and rituals – or they try to avoid it altogether, through procrastination, dropping out or drugs.

I'm guessing you are with me on this, right? You don't want an anxious kid? Or to raise an anxious young person? You want a brave, bold young person, who believes in themselves. So let me give you the heads-up here – it is not through your praise or their achievement that children get brave and bold; I have a whole stream of young people coming straight down from Oxbridge to my therapy room, riddled with self-doubt and full of fear. No, I think you get brave by not looking so much for those external baubles in life, and instead a growing sense of self-confidence in your own path, and knowing that you are going to be able to cope with and tolerate the mess along that path. Much of this comes down to an ability to bear uncertainty – not knowing what the future holds, accepting that we can't fully control it, and can be with it, whatever it is.[i] Balancing anxiety is sitting with the uncertainty that often requires a back-up of love and support from parents, who are also doing this.

So whilst it is normal to worry and constructive to feel fear sometimes, my second aim is for you to raise children who have a healthy level of anxiety and a tolerance for uncertainty.

Happyish young people

I also want our kids to have a capacity for joy. Too many children, adolescents and young people are spending their lives hopeless and utterly miserable. Some of them are so sad that they are self-harming, and some are so sad that they want to die. As with the concept of self-esteem, the idea of building resilience has been tossed around in child raising over the last generation and yet we have sky-high rates of depression amongst young people. And they are kind of being criticised for not being resilient enough, being labelled 'snowflakes'. I don't think they are not resilient; I think we, the adults, put them in too many situations that make them sad. It has happened on our watch.

The third aim is therefore to raise happyish young people. As with anxiety, it is not reasonable or realistic to be happy all the time. Indeed, that would be quite mad. If my dear dog, Suki, were to die today, it would be right and proper for me to be sad.[1] Were I happy, you'd rightly think I was uncaring or that I was a psychopath. But we want to raise kids who are happy enough to get through adolescence without cutting their arms – kids who can see the joy in life, the humour in darkness and the light at the end of the tunnel.

Relationships

Relationships are key to good mental health in adulthood. And key to good-enough relationships throughout life is the first attachment relationships a baby and toddler has with their parents. There are two aspects to these: the first is a sense of connection between parent and child, which will be a 'secure base' from which they can grow and develop; and the second is that this provides the internal infrastructure for children to hang other relationships on. Once kids have learnt about good-enough relationships through attachment, they have the capacity to do that in other relationships.

---

1 See my first book, *You Don't Understand Me*, for a photo of lovely Suki.

Throughout the book we will be returning to the things that enhance your relationship with your child, but if I had to pick one thing that is important it would be reciprocity. Too often, I see parents – lovely, kind, committed parents – who have become waylaid by an external agenda for their child or themselves: a busyness agenda, or a getting-on agenda or an appearance agenda. External agendas get in the way of seeing the child before you – and responding to them. Reciprocity gives you a good foundation for your relationship with them, but also gives them a good skill base for having relationships in the future.

Emotional competence

Our children live in a world that is infinitely more complex and stimulating than a generation ago. This, imho, has contributed to the mental distress of young people. To navigate this, we need to raise children who can regulate their emotions better than before, who show a degree of emotional competence that was not required in a slower, less connected world. This is my fifth manifesto aim. We need kids who are self-aware enough to recognise the impact of this complexity on them and have the emotional intelligence to navigate it. Emotional competence has lots of components, including a capacity to recognise and name your emotions, bring yourself back to equilibrium after a strong emotional reaction and to tolerate difference and take responsibility for this.

This is a tough gig for parents. There are many things that I suggest in this book that my own good-enough parents didn't have to do. Talking to a tween about avoiding internet porn, for example. Unprecedented times.

Independence

We want to get children to a point, preferably in their late teens or early twenties, where they are emotionally and practically capable of independence. We are trying to raise fully functioning grown-ups, who, to some extent, leave us and establish their own lives in which they can thrive. Because that is the purpose of parenting, right? I guess I pose it as a question because I see many parents who don't seem to act like that is their intention. They are or have been super involved in their child's life and want to continue to be so through adolescence and adulthood. They are not prepared to face their grown child's autonomy and wish to avoid the pain of the parent–child separation, which, in the long run, leaves everyone worse off.

I think we need to agree that independence is one of the manifesto outcomes . . . even if you are reading this when your child is a baby, or if they are at that really cute early-childhood phase when they promise you with wide eyes that they will never, ever leave you, and actually want to marry you. You need to keep your eye on the long-term ball, which is that you have to invest an enormous amount of time, money and your whole heart, for them to leave you behind and potentially do things you don't approve of and (here's the worst bit) for you no longer to be their primary relationship. For them not to love you best. The letting go might be one of the most painful bits of parenting: it might be like tearing a Band-Aid off your heart.

An older parent said to me when I had my first baby, 'You get an awful lot of teenager for a small amount of baby, so enjoy the baby bit'. That has always really helped me remember to find the joy in where I was at, and also in what I was losing as I was headed into the future. Now mine are in their late teens and early twenties, and on the cusp of leaving home, it feels that you get a relatively small amount of teenager, too.

So those are the six manifesto aims: the destination we want to get to with our children – where they think they are good enough;

that they should not be scared of life; that they can find the joy in it and regulate difficult emotions to help with this; and finally that they grow up and leave us, to develop new relationships, with our relationship intact. Through my studies, my work and in my home, that is what I have learnt about for the last thirty years, and it's what I'm going to share with you now.

MY FRAMEWORK FOR MODERN PARENTING

Over the last year, since I set out a manifesto and started to write this book, I've read hundreds of research articles and books; some old favourites and some new to me. I reflected on all my old patients over thirty years as a psychologist, and my own personal experience as a mum. I divided the book up into four development stages (babies, toddlers and pre-schoolers, children and then tweens and adolescents) and then dived into the issues at each stage. I wrote about 110,000 words, trying to make sense of it all, and then, you'll be very relieved to hear, I cut about 20,000 of them. I was trying to figure out what was key. What did we need to do upstream to achieve good mental health downstream?

As I was thinking and writing, everything kept coming back to three core things. They are:
- being a good-enough parent: not a neglectful one or a perfect one, but somewhere in the middle
- being a relationship-based parent
- being firm and kind in our parenting.

These three factors seem to be the crux of maximising manifesto aims and are, therefore, my framework for modern parenting. I'd like to say that I held this wisdom throughout my whole life as a parent and I planned the book around these points from the start. Sadly not. But I think they are important; no, not just important – key. Key to giving your child the best chance of a good-enough, happy life. They sound simple and, in a sense, they are. But there is certainly plenty more to say about them.

In a book that spans the eighteen years of childhood, I can't begin to cover all the issues you will face as a parent. So, I have picked out some specific ones – sleep, food, screens, school etc.– to illustrate how the framework plays out. On the other issues you will face? I do believe that if you come back to the framework, you won't go far wrong. Think of the three framework factors as the tripod legs holding up your parenting.

This book is based around general principles and rough stages, rather than specific advice or exact precision. It is structured around these four age-stages, but each bleeds into the others, so for example, stuff in the baby section is relevant to toddlers, childhood and teens, and the toddler section starts with stuff that is relevant to babies. One of the points of the book is to look upstream and downstream along the eighteen-year river: to understand how patterns and habits at one age are set up earlier, or impact a child later. I am going backwards and forwards in time; and I am talking about specific issues to illustrate general points.

There are also two chapters about you and your identity as a parent – at the great turning points of your parenting. The first is in the baby section and is about becoming a parent, and the other, in the adolescent section, is about letting your child go. I am sorry that these two chapters draw more on the maternal experience than the paternal – I draw on my observations of mums and dads, but my experience as a mum.

One more thing before we start: mental health is a continuum. On one end, we have mental wellbeing. When we are mentally well, we still experience ups and downs in our feelings, much as we suffer coughs and colds when we are basically physically well. Good mental health does not mean absence of difficult feelings. But on the other end, there is serious mental illness where, for example, people may lose contact with reality or become overwhelmed with thoughts and feelings that are out of proportion to any trigger event, prevent them from living life or last a long time.

Many of the factors I touch on in this book are about degrees: about maximising the chances to be at an optimal place on the continuum, or about stuff that might help move your child into a less suffering position. It is not the case that any factor 'causes' mental illness single-handedly. Mental ill health is more complex and nuanced than that and includes biological and genetic factors, as well as the parenting and societal factors that I am focusing on in this book.

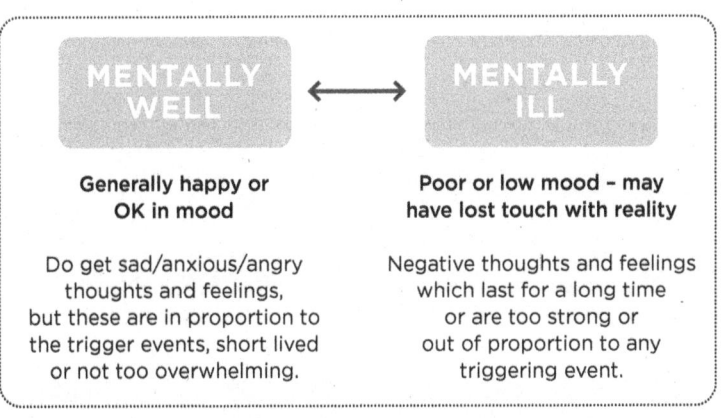

MENTALLY WELL ⟷ **MENTALLY ILL**

| Generally happy or OK in mood | Poor or low mood – may have lost touch with reality |

Do get sad/anxious/angry thoughts and feelings, but these are in proportion to the trigger events, short lived or not too overwhelming.

Negative thoughts and feelings which last for a long time or are too strong or out of proportion to any triggering event.

Where to start? With good enough, I think, because it is all-encompassing, in that you only need to be good enough on your relationship-based and firm-and-kind parenting. Good enough is, indeed, a good-enough place to start.

PART 1: BABIES

1.1
Starting Off Good Enough

When I write, I always try to imagine my reader. Who will be reading this book about being a parent? As it is about the whole of childhood, you might be at any stage: pregnant and thinking about how you are going to be as a parent; a relatively new parent of a baby or toddler, looking for guidance about sleep or tantrums. You may be in the hustle-bustle of the primary-school years, balancing so many different demands, constantly chasing your tail. Or possibly in teenage years, feeling exasperated and lost as to what to do; or in the empty-nest years, trying to make sense of it all. Of course, you may not be a parent at all; you may be reflecting instead on your experience of being parented. Parents are a thread that runs through all our lives.

You may be looking for answers to your parenting problems or someone to tell you what to do. I feel I need to be straight up with you: if you are looking for a parenting guru with all the answers, I'm not sure this is the book for you. I have been at the coalface of parenting and child psychology for thirty years, with a side hustle in the school system. I've learnt a lot about children, adolescents, parenting and education, and have boiled that experience down into this book. I have the manifesto to offer you and a framework to explore with you, but I simply do not have all the answers.

I also am wary of giving you a stick to beat yourself with, a standard to fail to reach, a story of the perfect parent that no one ever meets. Parenting has become big business. It's become an industry of selling stuff and self-improvement, and much of that is built on telling you how you are lacking. I do not want to do that. And I want to be honest with you, I am not a perfect parent. I have had all that experience with children, adolescence and parenting, but still cock it up on a daily basis. I fail to reach my own standards and expectations all the time.

Why? Because I am a human being in a relationship with my three children. I am not a computer programme or a piece of machinery. The things that make us human – things like thought, mood, personality, language and a capacity to relate – create an infinite amount of variability in our behaviour, and in the behaviour of others. There is no perfect because we are co-creating a relationship, in the space between them and us, and for that we need to see, hear and respond to the other person. Perfection is not a useful concept in relation to being human: there is no one right way to be; everything is a matter of opinion. And from variability spring meaning, creativity, joy, progress, humour. Aiming for your idea of perfection negates their (and your own) individuality: it would have us all the same and anything else inferior, or everything superficially positive with none of the difficult emotions. Yet to be seen and heard as ourselves is one of the most powerful parts of being human, and for a child to be valued and appreciated for who they are is one of the most amazing gifts a parent can give them.

Perhaps you are thinking, 'Well, I won't/don't expect my child to be perfect; I just expect them to be themselves. But that doesn't stop me being the perfect parent to that child, does it? I will be infinitely caring, endlessly supportive, constantly there for them...' Perhaps you believe that in this way you will achieve the manifesto aims outlined in the Introduction – that you will avoid your child growing up anxious or depressed? But I don't think so. I think if you aim for perfection, you will end up disappointing yourself, possibly having a miserable time and almost certainly setting your child up to be endlessly let down by the rest of life. Because, as we will see, perfect doesn't exist. Perfect is always chasing the end of the rainbow and never where you are. For this reason, the standard we should be aiming for is good enough.

I, I confess, am only and proudly a good-enough parent.

MY GOOD-ENOUGH CONTINUUM

Good enough is a big deal in the psychology of parenting. It was a concept first introduced in the 1950s by Donald Winnicott, a post-Freudian, British paediatrician turned psychoanalyst whose writings focused on the earliest part of life, grounded in his work with families, and particularly on the bond between mother and baby.[ii] The idea of good enough focuses on the everyday warmth and interactions between children and their parents and how these support children's psychological development.

Winnicott coined the phrase 'good enough' in his work seventy years ago, but what does it mean at this time to a modern parent? I think we need to think of a good-enough continuum. And start, at one end, with what good enough isn't. As a psychologist, I have arrived at home visits to find children climbing the walls, scrambling up the back of a sofa, precariously clasping a shelf with one hand, swinging across the room and their parents ignoring them as they watch the

TV with dead eyes. I have arrived to find a parent smashing their home up in anger, destroying the toilets, so the children can't stay there that night. I remember particularly the fearful, sad eyes of a four-year-old boy peeping from behind the curtain, as his mum spat vitriol about how bad he was. I have heard from adolescents and adults about being beaten, being ignored, being put into the cold, being neglected and being abused.

I think we can agree that all of this isn't good-enough parenting. We have one end of the continuum secured.

Many of the parents who committed these abuses had a history of trauma and abuse in their own lives. In addition, whilst I've seen this in all the different socioeconomic classes, for some parents it was linked to a lack of privilege: they were poor, alone and lonely, overwhelmed, undereducated or lacking in hope. Some had learning difficulties and/or physical and mental ill health. On the occasions I was working with them, I had to try to empathise with their backgrounds before I could help them move forwards with change, but this empathy was anchored in the understanding that this sort of parenting is not good enough. Abusive parenting is likely to exert harm – we may not know precisely what harm, but harm is likely. Contrary to the children's rhyme 'sticks and stones may break our bones, but words can never hurt us', research suggests the exact opposite is true: the toxic harm of the physical abuse is more in the meaning that children imbibe from it – the words in their head about the abuse, which are possibly 'this person doesn't love me'. This meaning can last a lifetime, long after the 'broken bones' mend.[iii] As these researchers put it: 'Emotional abuse emerged as the main independent predictor of psychiatric symptomatology over and above other maltreatment types'.

But swinging to the other end of the continuum, good enough doesn't mean you have to be a perfect parent either. The word parenting, positioned as a verb, as something active you do, rather than the word parent as a noun, you in relationship to your child, first emerged in books in the 1950s. From that time, being a parent was spoken about in terms of self-improvement, a skill you can learn, and with an increasing number of expectations.[iv] The parenting-as-a-verb concept really gathered momentum around the turn of the millennium: the parenting gurus, the TV shows, the pressure for parents to be constantly thinking about educating their children in play, word, and deed, the micro-analysis of every aspect of what we do to think about what is so-called best. The professionalisation of parenting as a full-time job.

I wonder if now we have reached peak parenting? I have certainly met a lot of parents who have given too much. Sometimes they are all about healthy eating: their child has only been fed only organic, sugar-free food, they think pasta is unhealthy and laugh at the mention of takeaway pizza as a possible dinner. Or their child is scheduled in a full range of creative, musical and physical activities from early in their first year, or, potentially worse, over-invested in one particular activity, which has become the linchpin around which their parents' lives are organised. Often, these days, parenting involves being active in securing their child's academic/economic future from birth: perhaps getting them into the 'best' school possible (for which read the one with the highest exam results). Parents move house or attend church to ensure this or tutor their kids through entrance exams. In the private sector, strings may be pulled, donations made, favours called in. Some parents channel their parenting drive into a planned, organised existence, Excel-spreadsheeted to within an inch of its life. For other parents it is all about having a perfect bond, being the all-giving parent, skin-to-skin touch or so-called 'attachment' parenting. Some poor kids have many of these different examples of perfect parenting imposed upon them. But whatever form it takes, parenting-as-a-verb, as opposed to being a parent in a relationship, is characterised by an attitude of self-improvement and striving.

It can feel as though parenting has become an extreme sport. In its worst iteration it has become a competition to create 'the best' child. Is this type of perfect parenting the good enough we are looking for? I don't think so. The potential hazards are less obvious, but I believe they are there. If one of your goals in being a parent is to raise children who feel good enough, your attempts to be a perfect parent may spectacularly backfire, instead embedding an expectation or a norm of perfection into your child's mind. Is that 'best'? In our race-to-the-top parenting have we unwittingly created a generation paralysed by perfectionistic standards?

I became alerted to this in my clinic, listening to mentally unwell young people, because many of them, whatever their official diagnosis, often don't feel good enough. At the core of their distress is this sense of helplessness as they try to reach high standards in multiple different dimensions, and, like juggling with a hundred balls, they just can't do it. They may be diagnosed with OCD, ADHD, anorexia, depression or pretty much any psychiatric condition, but underlying it is this feeling that they are not enough. Similarly, when I have seen anger and violence they often seem to spring from being overwhelmed or not valued: again, a sense of not being enough. A lot of the young people I see are achieving high grades, but they don't think they are smart enough. They are beautiful, but they don't think they are attractive or slim enough. They are funny and creative, but they think people don't like them.

They make the regional finals, but think they should make the national finals. They get A in one exam, but the next day feel a bit 'meh' because the relentless work schedule for the next one starts again. They hold a perfectionistic mindset whereby they are constantly striving for better and more. They never feel enough as they judge themselves constantly on multiple, shifting categories and so can always find themselves lacking somewhere. It seems this pervasive sense of not good enough is endemic to this time in history.

When I sit with these children and teenagers, I am often reminded of Jonny Wilkinson, the rugby superhero, who scored the winning drop kick in the dying minutes of the 2003 Rugby World Cup Final, securing the title for England. He has spoken about how achieving that degree of perfection with his drop-kick goals was achieved at the expense of his mental health. As he puts it, 'I lived a huge amount of my career thinking I was going to achieve joy through suffering'.[v] I worry that we are raising children by the same creed, and we are seeing the peak parenting attitudes reflected in the minds of our young people.

And this is what the research shows: that perfectionistic standards in parenting, education and society are not great for children.[vi] They can create a perfectionistic mindset in children and a vulnerability to mental-health problems.[vii] At one end of the continuum, we have solid research data about the long-term impact of abuse on children. Yet at the other we also have data that indicates that perfectionistic parents can also have a negative effect: there are lots of different paths along which this can play out and we will return to them throughout this book, but, for example, kids can internalise their parents' perfectionism or pick up on the associated anxiety; or parents' attitudes can warp the relationship between them.

Every day, I see so many children, adolescents and young people who are struggling, paralysed by the expectations on them or by an implicit assumption that they will reach or surpass their parents' achievements. Kids nowadays are surrounded by this striving, 'do-better-and-get-more' culture. Yet this generation are joining adulthood when the Western world is at a turning point, when, for perhaps the first time, a large swathe will likely be poorer than their parents. This creates a happiness gap: tech entrepreneur turned mental-health campaigner Mo Gawdat has analysed happiness and created an equation for it: happiness, he argues, equals your current reality minus your prior expectations.[viii] For parents and children raised with strong ideas about striving for perfection, this is a problem. Nothing about expectations of perfection prepares you for the hurly-burly life of secondary school, or getting a college job as a waitress, nor, quite frankly, compromising with other people in your close personal relationships.

So 'good-enough' parenting isn't the opposite of abusive parenting. Good enough is in the messy middle of the continuum, between abusive and this attempted perfection. I sometimes think of good enough as that place on a see-saw where you stand in the middle and are not jolted about by the extreme changes at either end. Finding balance in the middle isn't easy because you are constantly having to readjust. For this reason, good enough is not a cop out. It is a less certain state with a heap of compassionate self-reflection necessary to keep it steady. It is full of contradictions: you are going to have to be both consistent and flexible; to give lots of opportunities and have few expectations and, most importantly, mess it up and make it right again. But good enough definitely does not engage in some sort of competitive race to be the best parent or push your child towards any particular outcome.

GOOD ENOUGH IN BABYHOOD

Throughout this book, we will be returning to how good enough trumps perfect at the different stages of a child's life and on different issues, and what this means for you as a parent in practice. As you start out with a baby, good enough means that you can let go of a lot of preconceived standards – for yourself and for your baby.

Because standards are nearly always just a matter of opinion. For every parent who thinks that perfect parenting is skin-to-skin contact and feeding on demand, there is another who thinks it is all about getting the perfect routine and Gina Fording their baby into it. For so many aspects of parenting (or child 'outcome') there is not an agreed best. Any perceived perfection is only a moment in time, like Jonny Wilkinson's goal. Time moves on and something newer or shinier, or the next challenge or hurdle, emerges. One day the routine works perfectly, but the next, for no apparent reason it does not. As for my patients, getting an A on the test just means starting the slog towards the next: the perfect becomes immediately the past, either kind of irrelevant or a standard we have to try to meet again.

And whilst your newborn undoubtedly seems perfect to you, your job is not to keep them like that, like a china doll in a glass display. As American academic Brené Brown says in her famous Ted Talk on vulnerability:

> When you hold those perfect little babies in your arms, our job is not to say, 'Look at her, she's perfect. My job is just to keep her perfect – make sure she makes the tennis team by fifth grade and Yale by seventh.' That's not our job. Our job is to look and say, 'You know what? You're imperfect, and you're wired for struggle, but you are worthy of love and belonging.'

Your good-enough parenting is a compassionate place for you and your baby. It's not trying to shoehorn you or them into some preconceived notion or other person's beliefs. 'My baby isn't hungry now – oh well, they can have a bottle later; bloody hell, the house is a mess – how precious I used to be! But I'm knackered and enjoying cuddling my baby. That's good enough.'

Perfect parenting, in contrast, is an anxious state of trying to achieve: 'I should be breastfeeding, and giving my baby skin-on-skin contact, but my baby won't feed; and look at the house, it's such a mess . . . I hate it when it is messy; and I'm making myself late, and everyone else gets there on time – they are going to think I'm rubbish; and why won't my baby feed? I'm failing at this . . .'

Letting go of perfect standards can help us let go of that anxiety; and, to state the obvious, no kid wants an anxious parent. Anxiety can undermine relationships and spread rapidly. When you are anxious, there is a tensing up of your muscles, a quickening of your breathing, an increase of your heart rate. Your baby will feel that and, as they grow through the next stages of life, you risk them seeing all the dangers and problems that you see. They will learn, by example, to be anxious. We've all been around someone anxious and stressy, right? Panicking about whether you are all going to make the train, or whether they left the window open. And you've likely had the experience of feeling perfectly calm about it all, until they started stressing, so that ten minutes later you are worked up, too. Well, the same applies to you and your child: anxiety can be contagious.

Now, if you are of an anxious bent, you may be thinking that knowing this makes it worse, as now you are going to be anxious about being anxious. To that I would say this is not something to beat yourself up about – 'Oh God, I'm anxious and the baby knows'. It is a place to examine your expectations of yourself, then breathe and *let go of them*. Your job is to show up imperfect in your relationship with your baby. Being 'only' good enough is not letting yourself off the hook, or giving yourself a free ride; nor does it mean swinging to the other end of the continuum of being neglectful. In contrast, it actually means giving your child the very best start you can. In finding an imperfect middle ground, in the longer term you are giving your child the freedom to find their own path, rather than imposing your standards and expectations on them.

Good enough is clearly not neglecting your baby, but nor is it some sort of rigid routine you impose on yourself and feel guilty if you ever skip. Good enough is mostly being there for your baby, but also allowing yourself to miss the bath or bedtime routine to have a drink and a laugh with your mates. Good enough is, of course, ensuring that your baby gets fed, but not killing yourself making sure every feed is breastfed or with skin-on-skin contact. It's recognising that not every mum and baby can breastfeed: maybe that's you and your baby, and that's OK. It's good enough. Through the first year, it is making sure your baby gets roughly the right macronutrients on a week-by-week basis, though not necessarily at every meal. It's neither denying your child all sweets and chocolates, nor feeding them fizzy drinks and crisps for breakfast. It is neither strapping your baby to yourself for twenty-four hours a day, nor hiring a night nurse and day nanny so you can skip back off to your pre-baby life. It is somewhere in the middle of these extremes: it is about being responsive to your baby's needs but not dominated by them.

You see, Winnicott – the big-cheese psychotherapist who first spoke about good enough (see p. 19) – thought that in the imperfection of good enough a baby's brain learns to cope with real life, which is often unpredictable and imperfect. When you miss part of the routine, or don't breastfeed exclusively, or your baby is unsettled because you stayed out late laughing with your friends, your baby is still learning important things. They are learning about change, difference and flexibility. A baby needs to firstly have the experience of being cared for, of having placed inside them a nugget of core love, through a good-enough, responsive parent, but then over time they also need to learn to cope with not having all their whims catered to 24/7. Most of all, a baby doesn't need the parental expectation that they can be moulded into a perfect child, which is often a version of a parent's lost dreams. As psychiatrist Carl Jung said, 'The greatest burden a child must bear is the unlived life of its parents'.[ix]

When you, as a parent, meet your baby, it is like you are given an unmarked packet of seeds. You plant a seed in your garden, but you have no idea what it is. It may be a cactus, spiky and needing little water from you. It could be an orchid needing damp conditions, only flowering occasionally. Or it may be a tall, hardy tree or a delicate violet. You don't get to decide what they are, but the joy and challenge of parenting is working out what they need and then watching them grow as you adapt to their needs. You should neither trample on their growth, nor try to make them conform to the shape of other plants. Lots of parents are given a packet of seeds that are a bit like them – often, the apple doesn't fall far from the tree. But many receive an entirely different species of plant from them.

Most of all good-enough parenting, for me, is about an attitude. It is about letting go of your anxiety about reaching any standard for you or outcome for them, and instead putting your relationship with this growing individual at the centre of your world. It is an attitude that is freeing to you and to them. It is accepting that your power over their outcome is limited and, as with any power, it can be toxic and needs to be used mindfully, sparingly, judiciously.[2] It is accepting that, from birth, they are not 'tabula rasa', a blank slate – they come with their own innate characteristics and talents, which are likely to be different from yours – and doing the difficult task of valuing and accepting difference in another human being.

---

[2] If you are interested in this idea, check out Dr Russell Barkley's YouTube video where he talks about parents being shepherds caring for their unique children, not engineers designing them.

1.2
Relationship-Based Parenting

At the end of the last chapter I mentioned that part of good-enough parenting is putting your relationship with your child at the centre of your world, but not their outcome or progress. This is the second of the three elements of my framework for parenting: what I call relationship-based parenting. Again, through the book, we will be thinking about what this means at the different life stages, and here we start with the baby stage. There are so many competing demands on a new parent's time and attention – getting feeding and sleeping 'right', for example, or, indeed, getting dressed and out of bed at all. I hesitate to give you more to think about, but humour me as I explain why I think relationship-based parenting is important, and how to get that started.

ATTACHMENT THEORY
Attachment is the name given to the particular bond between a baby and their parent, which research and theory suggest has long-term consequences for a child's psychological development, and also forms the blueprint for all their future relationships. In previous generations, the importance of this relationship was

not understood at all.³ For example, in the past, children were routinely separated from their parents when they were in hospital. It was British psychiatrist John Bowlby who first observed the significance of the bond from his work as a psychiatrist with children separated from their parents during and after the Second World War, and the damage it did to them. His thoughts were later backed up with a whole heap of observations and experiments with animals, and by the seminal research of American–Canadian developmental psychologist Mary Ainsworth, where she studied babies' and toddlers' reactions to being separated from and then reunited with their primary caregiver.

At the crux of the theory is the idea that a baby is born looking to attach to a caregiver, and form a mutually satisfying bond that maintains the proximity between baby and parent. From an evolutionary perspective it makes perfect sense. Babies need someone to provide food and water and protect them from predators. But this bond is about more than just basic survival: babies seek warmth and affection and, generally, parents are drawn to provide it.

Experiments with baby monkeys carried out by American psychologist Harry Harlow at the University of Wisconsin–Madison in the 1950s illustrate the need for comfort. The baby monkeys were removed from their mothers and given a wire toy 'mum' linked to a bottle, and a soft toy 'mum' without food. A pure survival hypothesis to explain attachment would have assumed that the baby monkeys would have

---

3 I think lots of mothers (as the primary caregivers) did understand this implicitly, but in previous generations there was no research (or perhaps male appreciation) of this, and thus mothers and babies were forced into situations where their instincts were ignored. Traditional gender roles did not encourage men to be in touch with those instincts either, to be fair to them.

made a bond with the wire 'mum' linked to the bottle; in fact, they visited that one for food, but clung to the soft 'mum' for comfort. The photo below, showing the baby monkey clinging to his soft-mum substitute whilst reaching for food, so clearly demonstrates the need for comfort us mammals have.

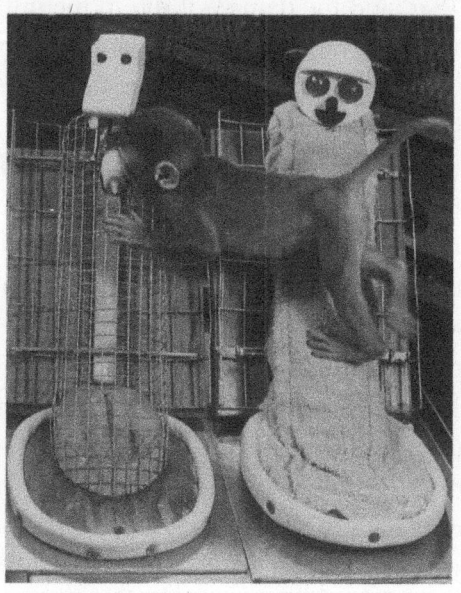

A quick note on gender before we go on. For historical reasons, in a less equal society, most of the research has been done with mothers, but babies are gender blind when it comes to an attachment relationship. Again, animal studies indicate this most vividly. Austrian zoologist and ethologist Konrad Lorenz showed how baby ducks will follow the first moving thing they see and think it's their 'parent' – in his experiments a wellington boot. Babies just want someone to show up for them. However, I sometimes use gendered language here, as society often does put pressure on women to comply with particular standards.

One of the many extraordinary things research has shown us about the significance of the attachment relationship is that a lot of its power and consequence take place in the baby years. We often think of relationships as linked to talking, but before your baby even develops any language, when you are still in the goo-goo-gah-gah stage of parenting, your relationship with them – or its absence – will form a long shadow in their psyche. Much of the research into this comes from studying adoption, and particularly looking at babies who are raised in orphanages before they are adopted. Orphanages are different from parents or foster families because they do not provide a chance for babies to develop one-to-one relationships, as there is a rotating cast of shift workers caring for them each day. Comparing orphanages from around the world has also provided interesting data, as they vary in quality, often depending on the stability or economic state of the country they are in. Research also compares babies adopted at different ages to different situations.

Unpicking this multitude of factors has proved fruitful to researchers. The consensus now is that experiencing individualised relationships in the first eighteen months of life is crucial for mental wellbeing later in life.[x] Babies who don't have this end up more likely to have social, emotional and behavioural problems later on, even if they've been well treated in their orphanage. Without this one-to-one relationship, there is some evidence that a baby's central nervous system develops to be hyper alert. Or, to put it the other way round, through attachment with a primary caregiver, babies are 'wired' correctly: the early one-to-one care creates the brain connections of trust, reciprocity and warmth, which are then in place for the rest of that child's life. When a baby has multiple caregivers they don't seem to develop this, however good the care.

As a parent it can be easy to dismiss the needs of a newborn baby: caring for one can feel like a boring, frustrating or relentless task and that you are just getting through the day. That feeling is heightened because, at first, your baby will appear to have 'indiscriminate attachment' and seem perfectly happy regardless of who comforts and plays with them. But actually, what you are doing by being there is forming that attachment bond between you and them: slowly, slowly, by showing up again and again, lifting, feeding, smiling, changing, tickling and chatting. And, with this bond, you are creating the blueprint for their future relationships, giving their brain the infrastructure for relating. By you showing up, even if they don't seem to recognise you, they learn what a relationship is about.

It is only in the second six months of life that a baby starts to show those signs of recognition. They get it: you are their person. In psychological language, they form 'a preferred attachment figure' who they look to the most, as a result of that person having been the one to have cared for them the most. In the second year of life they expand this to a hierarchy where a few attachment relationships emerge. This hierarchy does not seem to be about the strength of your relationship in the future: if a couple decide that one of them is doing the majority of the care and the other is working, it does not mean that in the future the child will always have a 'better' relationship with the attachment parent. Your future relationship with them will be more complex than this, depending more on temperament, interests, personality match. But a good attachment is about giving them a capacity to relate well with people in the future generally and future emotional stability.

For many, attachment may come easy: you may naturally feel a bond with your baby and hoover up the hours together.

For others, not so much, but don't despair. Because whether you find this early parenting a pleasure or a chore, if you recognise it is important, you can still do a great job. We often think about relationships in terms of what we feel, and, of course, what we feel is generally important in determining who you want to have a relationship with. But in reality, good relationships are not just about what you feel; they are more about what you put in the space between you and that other person. You may love babies, and delight in taking care of them, and that is great if you do. But not everyone does, and that is OK, too; you can still give attuned care in babyhood. You can give your kid a fantastic attachment experience by putting good stuff in that space, even if you sometimes find it boring or frustrating.

I like Katherine May's account of bonding with her son, Bert, in her book *The Electricity of Every Living Thing*. This book is an account of how Katherine discovered and came to terms with herself as having autistic spectrum disorder, and the difficulties with social interaction that she had to overcome in her life because of that.[4] For Katherine, her social difficulties are experienced in part as a sensation of electricity coming off others that earths through her, jolting her and exhausting her in the process. In the book, she recounts how difficulties with lights, noises and physical contact, and her need for a great deal of time alone, made her worry about being a good mother. But by the end of the book, she reflects on how she and her son (aged three at the time) have found an easy way to be with each other, snuggled up together in bed. She reflects:

---

4 The word generally used for this is 'masking': some people on the spectrum, particularly women, hide a great deal of sadness, anxiety and feelings of overwhelm inside of them, to act 'normally' on the surface.

And I realise, quite unexpectedly, that Bert is the only person in my life whose electricity exactly matches my own, whose touch is as native to my skin as air or water. There was a time when I couldn't bear this, when I wanted to be separate from him. That has passed. We have negotiated, between us, some kind of balance. I admire his patience with me, his willingness to adapt. But then I admire, too, my own adaptations. I begin to believe I am not so terrible after all.[xi]

What I love about this account is that it captures how it doesn't have to be quick, easy and natural; it can be a hard but no less important thing to build that relationship with your baby or child. Something that is in sync and reciprocal to your own kid. The first couple of years are important, but this is a marathon, not a sprint. It seems that a huge part of being a relationship-based parent is in the showing up and putting something good enough in that relationship space. Yep, even in relationship-based parenting you only need to be good enough; that's why good enough came first.

You don't need to be perfect. You don't need to be there all the time. Indeed, it seems the best sort of secure attachment is built not just on the being there, but also on the not being there. To understand this, I want you to put down the book and google 'Still Face Experiment' in videos. You should find something by Dr Ed Tronick. In the first part of the video, we get a brilliant illustration of how a relationship can be pre-verbal, as we see a mum goo-goo-gah-gah-ing with her baby of about a year. In the second part of the video, the mum stops interacting with her baby, and looks ahead with a blank expression. The baby works really hard to re-engage the mum, smiling, pointing, watching, and then becomes distressed. In the final part of the video, the baby is comforted by her mum re-engaging with her.

This video shows us three important things: in the first part, we see a good example of relationship-based parenting. This isn't big or clever, but what it is is *reciprocal*, where mum and baby are responding to each other. They are making eye contact, smiling, copying each other. They are putting joy and love in the space between them. A sensitive parent will be picking up their child's need for downtime, too; when the baby looks away or doesn't want to play or learn. It means accepting and responding to the child in front of you – not the child you wished you had; not the child you were and what you missed; not your pet project – not trying to reach superhuman standards of parenting.

The second thing we can see in this video is just how important this interaction is to the baby; and how she will work hard to get it. This matters to her. She is trying out her little tricks, the pointing and smiling that worked before to get Mum's attention, scanning her mum's face, looking for any reaction, and she is quickly not happy when she doesn't get one. The baby is wired to interact. I have used this video a lot in teaching, and it is this part that seems to surprise and upset my adult audiences: as the baby's face falls into distress, so do the faces of my audience. People have often spoken of feeling guilty about the times they have ignored their children seeing this. They don't need to feel guilty, though. And that is because of the concept of rupture and repair, which we see in the third part of the video.

RUPTURE AND REPAIR

When Mum joins in again, the baby is quickly soothed and comforted. Babies learn about relationships, not just through the interactions but through the 'rupture and repair' in these interactions. By rupture, I don't mean a baby crying all night, or being treated harshly or roughly. But I do mean the gaps that naturally happen in everyday life, when you are doing other stuff, and your baby learns that you are there for them, but increasingly you might not be there for them immediately. They learn to tolerate the 'separation' of being sat in their highchair whilst you are cooking a meal, or when they spend time being cared for by others whilst you get on with your work, or, perhaps most importantly of all, doing stuff that nurtures you. Then you come back: and you zone into them again. There we go, there's Mum or Dad, loving me, talking to me, responding to me. They learn that that is the pattern. These mini ruptures seem to work that attachment muscle more than simply being literally next to each other day and night. Rupture and repair might be a bit like the reps of weight training: it's not just the lifting of the weights that is important, it is the recovery time between weights, and the return for the next set, that build the attachment muscle.

Indeed, in these ruptures, your baby learns something really important about relationships, too. They learn about the imperfection of the world. They learn, in time, to self-soothe. They learn that other people are separate beings who they have to wait for, think about and negotiate with. This attachment blueprint you are putting down for them sets their expectations for other relationships not to be perfect.

So, what if these mini ruptures didn't exist? If you tried to be the perfect parent, always there for your baby, what then? There are proponents of twenty-four-hour parent–baby bonding who would say you have the baby in your bed, carry them in a papoose close to your heartbeat during the day. They would be steeped in this same attachment theory and would argue that it is a natural way to parent, arguing that through millennia women have strapped babies to their chests and got on with their work. I am a bit sceptical and wonder whether this is a romanticisation of the past . . . I'm guessing in the past women didn't use to be 100 per cent responsive to their kids all the time. My granny used to tell a story about leaving my mum and her brother in a tea chest, as she had to work on the farm sorting eggs during the Second World War. She didn't have disposable nappies or a washing machine. I'd imagine that under those sorts of circumstances lots of women weren't really attachment parenting – they were surviving.

I digress. I guess what I think a baby is learning from the twenty-four-hour-contact style of parenting is that someone is always there next to them. Deep in the brain of the baby, paths are being laid down for having constant comfort and their demands met immediately. Now, babyhood is all about giving a secure base of love that inoculates a growing child against the slings and arrows of life. But in my opinion, it is also about the slow growing apart of baby and parent, and I'm not sure that twenty-four-hour parenting is part of this process; rather, it cements the expectation that their parent will be there for them.

If you choose the twenty-four-hour style of parenting, inevitably, one day, there is going to be a time when you absolutely have to be apart – for you to get essential dentistry, for example, or to visit someone else you love in hospital. This may be difficult for you and your baby if you haven't previously strengthened their being-apart muscle. My prejudice from my clinical work is that sometimes this plays out as being a needy and demanding older child – an adolescent who phones their parent thirty times a day, unable to tolerate any distress independently. I say prejudice because, of course, it is only when it doesn't work that a child psychologist is consulted, but I'm sure there are children and parents for whom it does work.

STARTING YOUR RELATIONSHIP-BASED PARENTING
I've often thought that 90 per cent of parenting is neither pretty nor clever: it's just showing up. You don't have to give your all; you don't have to get everything right; you are allowed time off, and indeed it seems that will help you to build a healthy relationship with your child, them to build a healthy relationship blueprint for the future and build the capacity to tolerate your absence.

I think attachment is best thought of as a dance through life with your child: with you co-ordinating your moves to their cues. At this stage, you are mostly holding them in your arms, or their plump little hand, sing-song-singing with exaggerated mouth moves, rhythmical head moves and a bouncing knee action. But sometimes, you sit them on the edge of the dance floor in their little baby chair, as you dance with someone else, or on your own. You keep an eye out for danger, and for their distress, then you come and claim them into your arms again. A relationship-based parent isn't looking for a perfect dance. They aren't trying to shoehorn stimulation or learning into every move. They are offering instead synchronicity and empathy, and that often means meeting their child where they are at.

Ultimately, what a secure attachment in babyhood gives, what its purpose is, is to give children a sense of mattering through having someone strong and reliable who has shown up for them again and again. As babies, they will understand this unconsciously and implicitly; as they get older, they will more explicitly understand that you are there in the background if they need you, but also that they can cope and manage by themselves. That's your job: to give them that secure attachment at baby stage and then to gradually wean them off needing it so intensely during childhood, so that later a more adult-to-adult relationship can emerge. This is the crux of your relationship-based parenting.

1.3
Firm and Kind

So far we have covered two legs of the parenting tripod: being good enough and being a relationship-based parent. The third leg is what I call 'firm-and-kind' parenting. This is a style of parenting characterised by warmth, responsiveness, supervision and guidance, and in the psychological research it emerges with the best outcomes for kids.[5] [xii, xiii] We will return again and again throughout the book to this trio of parenting gold – good enough, relationship and firm and kind – and explore what they look like at the different stages as your child grows.

At the start of their life, firm isn't much relevant – being with a baby is very much about being kind – but one way it plays out is with sleep. As a child psychologist, you end up hearing about sleep quite a lot. Obviously, we receive training about it, and it comes up in nearly every case we work on. Sleep is fundamental to mental health, and how their children and adolescents sleep is a preoccupation of parents, often because it impacts on

---

[5] In the research, this style of parenting is called authoritative, which is a word that causes much confusion both because it implies the firm side of things is most important and because it is confused with a different style of parenting called authoritarian.

their own sleep – and without sleep everyone quickly ends up feeling quite crazy. For sleep difficulties in babies, sleep training is often recommended as the best treatment method. This is based on one of the main theoretical models in psychology: behaviourism.

BEHAVIOUR THEORY AND MANAGEMENT

Behaviourism emerged over a century ago and was a change of direction in the field of psychology. The word psychology derives from Ancient Greek, 'psyche' meaning soul, and 'logia' study, and from when the word psychology was first used around 500 years ago, until the behaviourism movement emerged at the turn of the twentieth century, it was used in reference to that which, at the time, was wholly unobservable, the study of the mind, brain, thoughts and feelings.

The early behavioural psychologists, such as Thorndike, Pavlov and Skinner, wanted to position psychology as a science with the same gravitas as chemistry or physics, and so advocated that psychologists should restrict their study to observable phenomena such as behaviour and action, rather than the unobservable feelings and thoughts. Behavioural psychology moved towards animal experiments in a lab, and a chasm opened up between this and the psychoanalytical schools of Freud and Klein, who were interested, in contrast, in focusing on clinical experience and unconscious phenomena.

Experiments looked at the learning schedules of animals based on providing or removing 'rewards' (things the animal wanted – largely food) or 'punishment' (for example, electric shocks) to train them. Watson and Skinner found that the animals, mainly rats, would learn through trial and error to press a lever to access food or to avoid an electric shock. Pavlov worked with dogs and found that when a buzzer noise came before food, over time, the dogs' salivation reflex was triggered by the buzzer. The early behavioural psychologists minimised the differences between animal and human psychology and hypothesised that humans would be subject to the same environmental learning as animals. For the behavioural psychologists, the newborn baby was seen more as a blank canvas that would be shaped by its learning experiences: the 'rewards' and 'punishments' (negative consequences) they received would determine its subsequent behaviour.

Simply, behavioural theory would state that any behaviour that produces a satisfying effect for a child is more likely to occur again in that situation. Parental attention, particularly warm and positive attention for stuff we want our kids to do, is the highest currency in this theory. And indeed, there is some truth in this: we know babies and children want attention because it confirms the attachment bond, which they are biologically programmed to maintain. In parenting work, I often describe attention as being like a miner's lamp on your forehead. What are you going to shine the light on? Stuff that you want them to do, and stuff they already do that you want to do more of.[6] The trouble with this is that often, as parents, we are busy getting on with life and only look and shine our parental light when we are interrupted by the sort of behaviour we *don't* want to see – bickering, fighting, moaning – and inadvertently end up reinforcing the bad stuff.

Sleep training emerges from behavioural theory with the logic that if you always respond to your baby's cries, they will cry more to get you to come, and not learn to settle themselves.

---

6 Thank you to my wise and wonderful previous supervisor, Jacqueline Byrne, for that one.

With its roots in the behavioural perspective, sleep training doesn't reflect on the internal world of the baby too much, but if it did, it would likely posit that crying is sometimes part of the falling-asleep process for a baby and does not mean they are upset.

The behaviourists see consistency as crucial, as otherwise, they hypothesise, you risk setting up a very sexily named 'partial reinforcement schedule'. This is when a baby or child gets a reward occasionally but not every time they behave in a particular way. An analogy is often made with gambling – people get hooked on gambling as they are craving that next win. In the context of babies' and small children's sleep, the behaviourists would say that if we 'give in' just one time and go to comfort them when they wake up, they are more likely to wake again, as they will want that 'reward' again. This is certainly not seen as a conscious decision by the baby; it is an automatic response to them wanting parental attention. It is a moot point at what stage in a child's development we would see it becoming part of some deliberate action by the child, but either way, the behaviourist would advocate giving minimal attention for sleep non-compliance and maximum attention and rewards for good sleep behaviour.

What I've learnt from my own experience as a parent? It's not that simple.

MY JOURNEY TO BECOMING A WORSE BEHAVIOURIST – PART I

When I was first pregnant, I worked in a psychiatric hospital for kids in central London. So many of these children had terrible sleep. Again and again, I would hear of horrible sleep routines in babyhood, which had morphed into co-sleeping in the parental bed, advancing to a position of musical beds in the childhood years.

I was so clear in my mind that this wasn't going to happen to me. I was fully schooled in sleep training and the behaviourism ethos. I remembered my own formative training experience, as outlined in the Introduction, where my supervisor reflected on how sleep was the fault line on which he, as a parent, had become a worse psychologist – but I was not having a child sleep in my bed for ten years.

I remembered all those parents with rather more humility as I sat, paced, rocked and cradled that first colicky baby. I remembered them, as I was delusional with tiredness one night, racking my brains for a solution, thinking that if I threw him out of the window, that would stop the crying. Not thinking this in anger or with any intent, but genuinely problem solving in my head about what could possibly stop this crying noise that was simultaneously breaking my heart and driving me insane – anything to make it stop. He screamed and screamed and screamed for hours every day. And I hadn't slept. In daylight hours, I made rational lists of things to try: colic drops ✓ cranial osteopathy ✓ routine ✓ . . . But at night, wild solutions came to mind.

And a routine did really help, tbh. At that time, around the turn of the millennium, Gina Ford, a hardline baby sleep trainer, was everywhere. I really didn't like the tone of her book *The Contented Little Baby Book*, because I don't generally go for strict dictates and absolute standards and am naturally a bit of a cuddler. In contrast, this was about letting the baby cry it out, and waking the baby up at 7am, leaving a sense that if you were to lie in till 7:10 you had failed on the day. But I was desperate, almost hallucinatory. Gina Ford was a real Marmite figure in the middle-class, pregnancy-yoga world in which I lived: the co-sleeping, feed-on-demand, go-with-the-flow parents were more vocal in my neck of the woods. But I was scared by my professional experience about how that played out ten years down the line. And Gina worked like magic on my colicky son. We went from eight hours of screaming a day to almost none. It was like *he* had read the book – he seemed to want to wake up and eat and sleep exactly when she outlined and was infinitely happier. And I could sleep.

So baby number two a few years later? I was ready. I had this.

Baby number two suffered with reflux. Reflux is a condition where the cap on your stomach doesn't work properly and allows food content to come back into your oesophagus. What it means is that when you lay a baby down, burning stomach acid comes back up; and for my baby, it initially meant she choked and then was usually sick. She didn't scream like number one, but she was clearly in pain. If I lifted her up vertically, she stopped choking and would sleep. We saw a doctor, she was medicated for the reflux and against the acid, so the pain went away for her. But there was no Gina Fording this one. On one day, I tried putting her down to sleep thirty-two times, and thirty-two times she woke up – as you do, it seems, if the contents of your stomach come back up into your throat. So I held her upright, night and day, in a tag team with her father, for five months. All my hard-and-fast behavioural principles were abandoned, as she was in my bed every night, and I learnt to sleep sitting up. Her reflux gradually got better, the cap on the stomach must have matured and suddenly she was able to lie down. And despite having pretty much slept only in our arms for months, she confounded my previously held behavioural beliefs that she would never settle herself: She went like a lamb in her cot and slept through the night.

So by number three, I felt I not only had the knowledge as a psychologist, I also had the experience of two radically different sleep problems in my first two. And despite these, they were both good sleepers as the toddler and child they had become. I was still optimistic. Possibly smug.

My third child broke me with his sleep. At first, he was an easy baby. At night, he always settled well at 7 or 8pm, on his own, and during the day, sat happily in his chair, watching the antics of his brother and sister. He didn't get much attention: he was too good for that, and in any case, I was too busy with his brother and sister. He was basically on a bit of a routine that fitted round a nursery and then separate school run; around making the other children tea; their activities; their bedtimes. At night, I used to wake him up for a feed before I went to sleep, and because I had so little time with him in the day, I cuddled him that little bit longer than necessary; inhaled his warm, milky smell, nuzzling his soft head and kissing his neck. I broke the classic sleep-training rule in that he often fell asleep as I cuddled him, enjoying that time with my baby. However, I also knew that behavioural theory wasn't the be all and end all; after all, my second child had slept only in my arms for five months, and that hadn't stopped her sleeping independently.

Whether this was causal or coincidental, I will never know, but he was a horrible sleeper throughout his childhood. He was a child who would try to climb out of his cot as soon as he could, so we moved him into a bed quite young for safety. And it was then that the problems with his sleep started. He wanted to be cuddled to sleep from that point onwards. If I went out, he was a nightmare, getting out of bed repeatedly, driving any babysitter mad. Then he'd wake up in the night and need more settling.

This didn't worry me at first: I had a reasonable track record as a parent at this point: I'd got my colicky baby and my refluxy baby into good routines eventually. Also, I was a psychologist – this was bread-and-butter work for me! I'd invoke the behaviourist within me and put him back to bed, again and again, calmly and consistently, with no positive reinforcement (attention) for him. He, it seemed, was not a behaviourist. It made no difference. He continued to get out of bed, long after his brother and sister were needing to go to bed. I tried a different behavioural principle, gradually withdrawing my attention, sitting with him with a neutral face, and no attention, and then slowly moving further away from him every night. This had no impact. I used reward charts, designed especially for him and applied with the regularity and consistency of a German car. No change. I got hardline and would leave him upset. It didn't seem to make any difference. In short, I used all the techniques that I had heard my supervisor outline to exhausted, frazzled parents years before.

This was not only exhausting and annoying as a parent. It was affecting my self-worth as a child psychologist. How could I now be the frazzled parent? One night, he broke me, and I lost my temper, and in that temper, I threatened that he wouldn't get his Easter egg if he came downstairs again. This was not a nice thing to do (no shit, Sherlock). But also, it was not an effective thing to do, in that it didn't teach him to go to sleep on his own. I think it just taught him that Mum was sometimes mean.

When I'd calmed down, and went up to check on him, I found him asleep on the stairs. I felt my heart melt, and I realised that boundaries and behaviour management didn't always work and were only part of a very complex story. I knew that I had lost that battle. I just simply didn't want my child so scared of falling asleep on his own, for whatever unknowable reason, and too scared to come and find me because I was as mad as hell, that he fell asleep on the stairs. And whilst I'm sure the behavioural psychologists are right – that if I'd left him to cry long enough or hard enough, of course he would learn to settle himself – I didn't want my child to feel like this. Despite all my best efforts, my specialist knowledge, my patience and, eventually, my impatience, my child was telling me without words, 'I really, really, really don't want to go to sleep on my own, and I'd rather fall in an exhausted heap on the stairs than do that' – and I wanted to listen to that. So I cuddled him to sleep nearly every night until he was ten. It turned out that snuggling down in his bed, kissing his soft hair, breathing in his little-boy smell, was often the best part of my day. Then, when he was about ten, he decided one day that he no longer wanted that anymore, and that was it: that time of my life was over. Nowadays, he's taller than me, and cringes when I give him a kiss. I guess I'm glad I got a lot of kisses and snuggling in when I could.

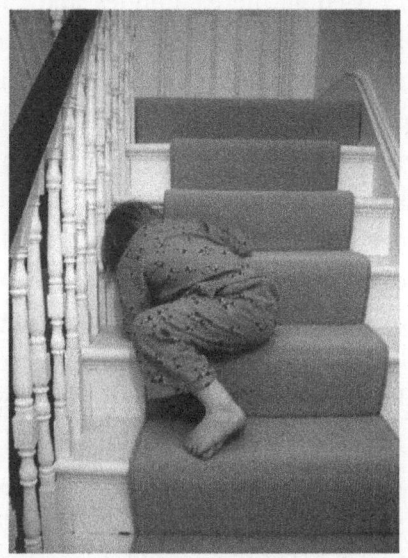

THE MESSY MIDDLE

What I learnt regarding the theory and research on sleep training vs the reality with my own children was fundamental to my ethos as a parent, and then, by extension, as a psychologist treating children and adolescents, and advising their parents. And I guess it's about that notion of a continuum of parenting, and that mostly the answer is found in the messy middle of the various conflicting theories and advice gurus. It is about compromise, trying things out, advance and retreat, consistency *and* changing your mind. It's not clear or simple. And it's about using the principles of firm and kind.

So what is the parent continuum on sleep? Well, on one side we have the hardline sleep trainers: leave them to cry it out. And they would state that they have some evidence on their side, which, if your outcome is wholly measured in short-term sleep gains, is pretty convincing.[7] [xiv]

But when, after many attempts of well-applied sleep training, I found my third child sleeping on the stairs, rather than coming to find me, I had a feeling that I was being a bit 'Romanian orphanage' in my parenting style, and that didn't feel comfortable.[8] You see, there's a difference between a little bit of controlled crying to train your baby to settle themselves, and children who stop crying because no one comes to them. And when I found my son asleep on the stairs, I had a flash of realisation that I didn't want him to feel like an abandoned child at bedtime – I wanted him to feel love. I really tried to be firm with my third, but firm then tipped into feeling mean, and I had to invoke kind instead. Firm and kind are both important, crucially important, all through your child's life, but if they get into battle, *choose kind every time.*

---

7   In chapter 2.1 on toddler tantrums, I'm going to go through why short-term research findings are sometimes not applicable to our lives as parents.

8   Under the regime of Ceaușescu in the 1980s, contraception and abortion were banned, poverty was rife and the orphanage population increased. In some of these orphanages, children were neglected or abused.

Because when you look at some of the behavioural studies, the principle of sleep training is based on dogs eventually stopping trying to escape the electric shocks that were being inflicted on them. They entered a stage called learned helplessness, where they gave up and, even when they could escape, they didn't. This feeling of learned helplessness is one of the characteristics, perhaps even the fundamental characteristic, of depression.

As a psychologist and a parent I often think about the developing brains of children and adolescents, and what new connections are being made by any situation. In sleep training, say if your baby cries a few nights, for an hour or two, they are making new brain connections of settling themselves, but if your baby or young child is crying for hours over weeks and weeks, I guess they are making a connection that you don't care.

So when I think about firm and kind and sleep, I also think about the relationship-based parenting that I outlined in the last chapter: responding to the kid in front of you and not the one in a parenting manual. The fact is that you and your child are both unique individuals who have to learn to rub along together. My first was colicky and needed the consistency of a routine. My second wouldn't sleep alone as she had reflux, but wasn't hooked on our attention, and happily settled when she wasn't in pain. And my third really hated sleeping alone, perhaps because, being the youngest, he had had less sense of attachment during the day than the other two, or perhaps not: we will never know. I'm guessing here, but with two others in tow, I bet I did less of the goo-goo-gah-gahing with him than I had with the others. But the point is: they were all different. My job as a parent isn't to impose my will over that according to some theory or ethos; it is to hear and see that, look at my own needs and capacity, and find the kindest compromise that is the best fit. That path, my friend, is often in the messy middle. And that is what being in a relationship is all about – and it is definitely good enough.

You may be reading this as the parent of an older child, teenager or adult, thinking, 'I got this wrong . . . I was too harsh/too overindulgent'. Well, I would say, so did I. But the path you start on doesn't determine where you end up. There is always time to change paths.

1.4
Your Identity as a Parent

> As we step into the new phases of our life, our identity will require ongoing negotiations.
>
> Julia Samuel, This Too Shall Pass

So that's your introduction to my tripod for holding up your parenting: to allow yourself to be good enough, to prioritise your relationship with your children and to have a firm-and-kind mindset. I want to pause here, in the baby phase, though, because there's one more thing that I think is really important – and that's you.

In many of the parenting books I've read, there is a lot about the nature of babies or children, and there is a lot about what you as a parent should do, how you should act, but there is less about you as a person. The focus is on children's behaviour and feelings and how you should respond as a parent – what *you* should *do* to manage *their* difficult emotions. There is less about your emotional reaction. There is often, I think, an assumption that parents 'act' with neutrality, rationality and wisdom, separate from their own psychological baggage.

With my framework for parenting, I guess I think we should do this a bit differently – because if you are practising relationship-based parenting, who you are is half the story. We are thinking about what you put in that space, rather than what you pull out of your child in terms of an outcome. This should, of course, be the good-enough, positive stuff, but it also has to be the genuine stuff. To be in a genuine relationship with someone you have to act with integrity in line with who you are. These statements might seem contradictory, as what if who you are naturally is someone who is grumpy or controlling (really, I see you)? Then, surely if you are acting with integrity, you are going to put grumpy and controlling stuff into that relationship space, not good-enough, positive stuff. Well, no, because you need to acknowledge your natural self and then reflect, grow up and put the best of yourself in that space. You have to embrace your emotional competence. That might mean turning the volume down on some bits of yourself and up on other bits. It needs thinking about because unexamined, unacknowledged feelings have a way of coming back to bite you, or worse, your children. Parenting isn't just a role you can act; it's a relationship you have to grow into.

As I have already confessed, I had all sorts of preconceptions and prejudices linked to my work, my social class and my own sense of self that I had to let go of to meet each of my children where they were. I had to see some of my own worst self before I could become the parent I ended up as.

That's why this chapter is about you, and your identity as a parent. Because your identity as a parent – how you are in your parent role – is the setting agent for all your parenting decisions. Your parenting will incorporate your ethos, beliefs and philosophies, your current social/emotional relationships and community, your history of being parented (and, by extension, your parents' history of being parented), your personality and mental health, as well as your wishes and dreams as a parent. Through all this, you bring your own stuff into raising your children. Thinking about yourself and how to put a good-enough but true version of this into your parenting relationship will help to establish a solid attachment that can pass down generations. Good attachment relationships are the ultimate family heirlooms, worth more than wealth or success. Your parental identity has a nemesis you have to watch, though – and that is not who you are but how-you-want-to-be-seen.

Whilst your identity as a parent will come up again and again in nearly every chapter of this book, there are going to be two separate chapters on this: one here and one after the adolescent section. These are the two times when your identity will be in flux: as you become a parent and as you start to step back from the active parenting to facilitate your adolescent's independence. In this chapter, nestled between the baby and toddler sections, we are going to look at how three aspects of a new parent's changed identity impacts on the framework for parenting. They are: how our work identities clash right into a baby's attachment requirements; how the change that becoming a parent brings can suck us into looking for certainty and control; and finally, how the insidiousness of the perfect parent, particularly from the internet, can worm its way in and undermine your good-enough parenting.

PARENTAL LIFE AND WORK
Up until a couple of generations ago, people were shown only one possible identity for their lives. Through church and state, almost the only path offered was to get married, have kids. More recently, parents have become older and more established

in their pre-baby lives, and there is more to lose in the decision to have a child. The loss of pre-child identity as an independent person, or an ambitious worker, or a sexy lover. Your new-parent role likely involves many changes to much of your previous existence, but perhaps the biggest threat is to your professional or work life. And this is a two-way street – because your professional or work life can undermine your attempts to be a relationship-based parent, too. Of course, work may not have been important to you, but if it is/was, it is likely it has to scooch over a bit to make room for the new parent you. This is the loss. You cannot do it all. Nobody can and nobody has.

Our attachment to our professional identity has likely been underpinned by two seismic changes that have happened in tertiary (post-eighteen) education over the last generations: the first is a worldwide increase in participation generally, from 8 per cent in 1970 to 45 per cent in 2022.[xv] The second is the proportion of women included in that figure: in the UK in 1970, 30.5 per cent of university students were women; by 2022, this had increased to 56 per cent.[xvi, xvii] My generation and since have been encouraged, taxed, socially shaped into degree-level education, two-parent working families and an expectation of consumer goods. As we have settled down to start our families, we have used our two incomes to outbid each other on houses, contributing to house-price rises and thus trapping ourselves in a reliance on two incomes rather than one.[xviii]

I'm going to bring you to my present in writing this: I am finding this next bit very hard to write. I am aware that, were I reading what I'm about to write twenty-four years ago, it might have felt like a threat to *my* identity as a feminist, my ambition in my career and my independence as a woman. Previously, the joy/sacrifice of looking after children and giving up career development has been all on women. Now, whilst that prejudice still exists, we are more equal than at any time in history. This is, imho, an excellent thing, but one that raises a difficult issue in that the type of care we've seen a baby needs is at odds with two working parents. Babies thrive with the kind of one-to-one, individualised care that, due to historical norms, threatens particularly women's autonomy and freedom. In short, it's best, early on, if all that potentially boring, repetitive stuff of feeding, nappy changing, goo-gah talk, putting them down for naps, etc. is done by a relatively small number of the same people, who can really develop an attuned relationship with the baby, pick up their social cues and be genuinely responsive to them. Attachment theory and research suggest that babies feel attached and calm, and learn to relate in the future, through one or two primary caregivers and not the excitement of new or less known people.[9]

This is an uncomfortable fact for many parents, including me, but one of my manifesto goals is emotional competence, and sitting with emotional discomfort is part of this. That involves the naming of difficult feelings and not rushing to rid oneself of them, but rather understanding them and making wise choices.

The research on childcare is a hornet's nest, often tied up in contradictions and institutional sexism. For example, much of the research in the past confused all non-maternal care with childcare – so if the baby was being taken care of by their father

---

9 I haven't come across any research looking at attachment in a situation where mums and dads are raising a baby with equal contribution; and of course, that would be difficult research to do, as, even if two parents are doing an equal amount of childcare, each one's style and relationship to the baby will be different. A baby is a human who has a preference for different styles, too – there isn't one 'right' style. However, my prediction would be that a baby would make two attachment relationships, in the way that a toddler raised in a dual language environment will learn two languages.

or grandparents, that was bundled together with childcare for research purposes, which makes no sense from an attachment perspective. In addition, there is confusion between interventionist childcare for deprived or struggling families and nursery care chosen often by professional, two-income families, which are obviously two very different things. The former is hypothesised to be putting the baby in a better situation than the home one; the latter assumed not. And there is also confusion about the word 'nursery' in the research, which can mean both early baby group care, and also means pre-school education for three- to four-year-olds; the needs of these two ages are very different.

There is substantive research showing that babies and toddlers have higher cortisol levels in childcare compared to when they are in home environments.[xix] On the other hand, there is equally substantive research showing that cognitive and academic outcomes are higher in the long term with group care in early years.[xx] So does that mean babies are stressed when they are little, but grow up a tad smarter? But there is also a lot of research suggesting that kids who spend longer in group childcare show, on average, marginally more behaviour problems later.[xxi]

I've read stacks of this research, and the following are, I think, the key points. Firstly, as babies, children need individualised care with someone they can get to know, and in group care that is likely less easy, as the very advantage of group care is that it is undertaken by a team, rather than one person. Secondly, whatever type of care you choose, quality is key: you are looking for lots of warm interactions between carers and babies. In reality, that can really only happen if whoever is looking after your child both really likes doing that and isn't looking after lots of other children, too. Inevitably, that is expensive, as it is trying to replicate the individualised care a baby would get in a good-enough home. There are sometimes calls to make childcare cheaper, but the only way we can do that is if we give an adult more babies to look after – say four or five – and this is counterproductive, as then they simply can't build one-to-one relationships, and will have less job satisfaction. Thirdly, as a parent you should be looking for fewer hours of group childcare early on, meaning fewer days but also shorter days. Finally, later on, at toddler age, group care, 'nursery school', can be a positive thing, especially for language and cognitive development.

What this raises for me, though, is the limits of a marginal-gains approach to parenting. Of course, research into child development is important, but if we pay too close attention to every marginal gain or benefit that some or other research shows that we can possibly give our baby or child, we are looking at one detail and not the whole picture. On childcare, the whole picture includes you and your partner, and a whole heap of other factors, like the availability of different childcare options in your family and local community. You are making your childcare decisions within that context, rather than that of the average baby from the research. Research tells us how most but not all respond. When we play the marginal-gains game, we risk forgetting to listen to the most important people: ourselves and our babies. Marginal gains parenting is the mentality of outcome- rather than relationship-based parenting: it is a striving mentality, rather than a flourishing one. When we think like this we end up painting by numbers instead of creating our own masterpiece.

As I said earlier, having a child is a marathon not a sprint. And it's a marathon that's likely to last the rest of your life. My view on a race of this length is that a) not everything will be perfect and b) if it were, it wouldn't prepare your kid for real life. Giving up your work, if you love it and need the money, to avoid the marginal disadvantages of group care for your baby, would be daft. You may end up bored or resentful and then you will not be offering good-quality care . . . back to square one. You know now babies need a lot of one-to-one interactions, and you want to use a nursery, so as a relationship-based parent you are going to need to figure your way through that, and make sure you make enough time and space for that goo-goo-gah-gah stuff to happen. It's a compromise, right? In the messy middle: it's not perfect. We are only two generations away from kids who were left in tea chests whilst their parents worked, remember: we want to be good enough; we are not aiming for some false notion of one-size-fits-all rightness or perfection.

Alternatively, you might love the baby stage, and not like your old job, and you might want to be a full-time parent. Let's sit with that for a moment, where you are loving having a baby and just want to suck up every minute of the deliciousness of your baby. I hear you. I love babies, too. Well, in one way that is great and fab, but in the spirit of emotional competence and sitting with the discomfort, I do just want to raise a couple of other issues. Sometimes a baby can provide an out. Sometimes, and of course not always, a baby provides a way to avoid something – for example, that you hate your job, or that you've not been as successful as you would have wanted. In a family where one parent hates their job or makes less money, it can completely make sense for them to give up their job to care for the baby – but their baby is not the long-term solution to that uncomfortable dilemma; to their feelings about their life trajectory.

And even if that isn't true for you, I still want you to keep an eye on your long-term future. In twenty years' time, that baby will be all grown up and likely to phone you once a week, if you are lucky – and that is right and proper. And in the medium term, they will be going off to school and wanting to hang out with their friends. There is a balance to be struck in raising your kids, between their life and future on the one hand, and yours on the other. One question here is how much are you willing to give? But another is how much is it helpful to give? I'm going to suggest you look after your future you not just because that is good for you, but also because it prevents you investing too much in your child and the risk of finding your purpose through their long-term need. Your job, as a parent, is to wean your children off needing you, not to cement that. So give up your previous life if that suits you, but never neglect your future self. You *and your children* need your future self. You are keeping an eye on your child's future independence and competence by keeping an eye on yourself.

When my kids were small, I kept on my fridge a quote from Christine Lagarde, who was Managing Director of the International Monetary Fund at the time. It said, 'You can have it all, but just not all at the same time'. To parent involves sacrifice: you will have to give up stuff to have time to form a relationship with your child, and, because of what a baby and child needs (i.e. you to show up), one of those sacrifices will likely be in your professional or work life. But you don't want to do this so much that you are resentful or fail to take care of yourself; nor so little that you don't meet their needs. Find that balance.

FINDING YOUR PLACE AS A PARENT

At the point when you have a baby, your identity changes – you become a parent, and you have to figure out what that means for you: what sort of parent are you going to be?

As we've seen, your professional identity may recede a bit, but in a hyper-visual consumer culture, there are plenty new potential identities waiting in the wings. We are not only sold prams, nursing bras or baby food, but also presented with competing philosophies and gurus of parenting and stacks of images of parenting. We also meet other new parents and, hopefully, start our parenting community. And because our old identity is somewhat battered and torn, along with our pelvic floors or abdomens, we are perhaps more swayable as new parents. With old relationships and roles in flux, and this new baby taking so much time and energy, you may wonder, who am I?

I spent a lot of time with my neighbour across the road when our firstborns were little. We hung out in parks, in our kitchens, in our back gardens. We swapped kids, so each of us could have our hair cut. We drank a lot of tea, ate leftover sausages and watched the clock for 6pm, to open the wine. We still do that, actually. We shared our parenting failures with each other, and often doubted our parenting styles. It seemed to us that other parents seemed more certain of what they were doing.

In one corner, we had the 'Tiger Mums': these parents had routines and boundaries, Gina Ford was well thumbed, the kids were neat and co-ordinated. They were on time. They were on time to a lot: to the parent-and-baby groups and swimming lessons, to Tumble Tots and Mini Mozart music classes. They had their child's name down for 'the best' schools or were strategising church attendance/catchment-area house moves.

In the second corner, we had the uber-relaxed parents – they were co-sleeping with their babies and breastfeeding. Conversations with them would be repeatedly interrupted by them paying intense attention to their child's every utterance. They didn't go in for too many formal activities, except, perhaps, baby massage. They were looking at Montessori nurseries and forest school.

We bemoaned our lack of an overriding ethos, and blamed our parenting failures on this. If our children were cheeky or disobedient, we berated our own failure to be strict like the Tiger Mums. We needed to give them routine! Activity! Structure! If, a week later, they cried with exhaustion after we'd dragged them round to Tumble Tots and junior basketball, we questioned our lack of patience. Why couldn't we just hang out with our kids, making dens and water play like the relaxed mums? Why were we carting them around all those activities, which made them tired and us harassed? Thus, we oscillated and fluctuated back and forth through their childhood, determining to be stricter one day and more lax the next. We looked at both camps with wonder and awe. How did they have so much certainty?

As I've progressed as a parent and a psychologist, I've come to wonder whether certainty was the panacea that I thought it was. I've come to believe that, as in many things in mental health, being in a balanced middle position is probably best.[10] I've come to recognise that flexibility and responsiveness are not necessarily weak or directionless, but actually allow for the child you are parenting, the life you have to lead and, of course, the growth and development of your child. They allow for a relationship to emerge between you and your child, where you are responsive to (but not dominated by) what they bring. I also have realised that people are drawn to certainty and extreme positions because it is more comfortable than balance. Balance is tough. It involves a constant state of readjustment. It involves questioning yourself; being vulnerable enough to ask, 'Have I got this right?' – and to change if you haven't.

As we look around this world, we see how, in human psychology, people are drawn to extreme positions as they provide clarity and certainty. We go down rabbit holes and stay down there – rabbit holes are comfortable and safe, and we find our

---

10 I'm not certain of this, obvs.

kind. As with parenting, it's psychologically easier in some ways to pick an ethos or group and stay there than to sit with the discomfort of uncertainty. But these competing ideologies offer false promises: there are no certainties in having a baby; you do not control their outcome or progress, whatever parenting style you use. Having a child is all about being able to embrace that vulnerability of love without control. As psychotherapist Cynthia Rousso says, 'I do not control my child's destiny'.[xxii]

So whilst it might be tempting to find a parenting identity that is clear cut and all in, I'm increasingly convinced that the best chance for kids' mental health when they grow up is not found in parental certainty and control, but in flexible consistency. We want them to be joyful, brave, flexible and emotionally competent, and those things are rarely found through parental rigidity. Instead, we are looking at the firm of clay and not the rigidity of steel. And that means you don't need to have your parenting identity figured out straight away; you can change and grow in the role, and in the relationship; and that meanwhile the messy middle is a good place to hang out. Most of all, you don't need to be perfect.

IDENTITY AND PERFECTION
I've already set out my stall on perfection in the 'Good Enough' chapter, about how putting a relentless quest for the 'best' into your relationship with your child will likely not benefit them. But I just want to have a think here about how and why you might be vulnerable to doing that as you become a new parent; and also how, if you do aim to be a perfect parent, it is insidious for you as well as your child.

Perhaps new mums have always taken the uncertainty of giving birth and the loss of their pre-child identity and tried to turn them into a perfect tableau of family and home. I'm thinking the 1950s' quintessential mum here. But has this been heightened by the current uber-commercial and internet-dominated society? You see so many images of 'perfect' mothering that can creep into your unconscious and impact your identity.

Of course, it is inevitable as a new parent that you will look around and compare yourself to other parents you know and parents in the media. Comparison is a natural process for humans. We can learn and grow through comparison – but were we designed to compare on the scale we currently do? Our innate urge to compare can't cope, for example, with Instagram – which is ironic, as it's probably human frailty that drove its creation.

Through comparison, stealthily and unconsciously, expectations of yourself can creep in. And like comparison, not all expectations are a bad thing. But here, it's about the sheer number of expectations and standards: the way you look, the way your home looks, the way your baby is dressed, the milestones they are meeting (or not), the work/childcare/breastfeeding dilemmas, the routine you follow, the food you give . . . You will be told tens of thousands of times, via advertising, that you 'must have' this 'essential' product. You will read daily in the media that this or that is (marginally) better for your child. You will inevitably absorb images and ideas of how parenting should look and be. And, if you are not careful, these will translate in your head into expectations of what you 'should' do or how family life 'ought to' look.

Have the internet and social media become a new version of what will the neighbours think, with the neighbours having become digitally and handheld, worldwide and there at every moment? What would people think? How does this look? As you compare your secret, messy life to a million images of 'better', inevitably, there will be a disparity between these expectations and you and your family. Your evil parenting nemesis – 'how-you-want-to-be-seen' – will come and fill this gap. And when he or she rears their head, you forget to be good enough, because they demand that you parent to the perceived standards of others. A false front: a triumph of appearance over substance.

I see this in my teenage and young-adult patients all the time, taking a third-person stance on their own life: thinking less 'What do *I* think and feel?' and more 'What do *they* think about me?' A focus on appearance and outcome encourages a viewing of yourself as a product, imagining yourself constantly reviewed on Person (Parent?)-Advisor, a fantasy about other people's opinions of you taking place in your own head.

New parents are subject to this same pressure because, like teenagers, their identities are in flux. There is, for example, a super-smug internet meme going round at the moment saying, 'You only get eighteen summers' – usually accompanying sepia-edged photos of smocked-dressed cuties running on the beach. They are trying to sell you the smock or the beach or an ethos of parenting. But they are doing that by selling you an image of perfection that, I think, can get in the way of you developing your own identity as a good-enough parent.

Because those eighteen summers you get with your kid are likely to include, in reality, snotty noses on sandy faces, someone getting sunburn, someone having lost their hat . . . Over eighteen years, someone will undoubtedly get ill, flights will be cancelled and there won't be enough seats as you wait at the airport. Someone will push someone else, and their ice cream will fall in the sand, and they will cry or punch their sibling back. It's likely you will lose your sense of humour, shout and give random punishments that you will never follow through with. You will do this and feel as though you are failing, and that, I think, will be exacerbated by the fact that, unlike other generations, you will have an expectation of how it *should* look in your mind, having seen thousands of images of perfect parenting. None of this will look like that internet meme.

Because there she is in your head, the internet-perfect-parent, calm, attractive, serene, with her compliant, beautifully dressed children instantly available for you to compare yourself to; to make you feel inferior. To make you feel not good enough. And what will you do with that feeling? Well, you are likely to want to be rid of it pretty quickly. You don't want to feel you are getting it wrong (you don't want to be seen to be getting it wrong). You've given everything to your parenting: you've read all those parenting books; you've made so many sacrifices. Don't they know how much you've given? Why won't they just behave? What is wrong with them? Your perceived 'failure' in your own mind is perhaps projected on to someone else – maybe your kids? Maybe your partner? – to protect your internal, wished-for perfect-parent identity. The martyr mother, giving so much; the best mother ever, famed from so many Mother's Day cards. Or the strong father; leading the family; listened to and respected. Cue the sense-of-humour failure, the snapping at kids being kids, the incapacity to relax, to let things just be, to enjoy the moment.

That feeling can, in time, breed a passive-aggressive, potentially controlling resentment. Anyone know a parent like that?

We can get so wedded to our image of ourselves that we forget that it is the doing and being a parent that matters. The image of ourselves, that we try to present to the world – the wanting to be seen as a perfect parent – can be our downfall and can very much get in the way of being a good-enough one.

When our children are little, our expectations can make us resentful when they don't sleep to our sleep schedule or mess our homes. In terms of my manifesto, it prevents us from modelling emotional competence, of literally and metaphorically sitting with the mess and accepting the good-enough life. It gets in the way of joy, as we are too busy tidying and putting on our make-up, and it puts us under pressure time-wise. It makes us anxious, as we are preoccupied with other people's judgments, and that anxiety is highly infectious for our children. It stops us seeing who they are and what they are feeling, as we are too focused on what it looks like, and that means we aren't relating. There is an irony that aiming for perfection in yourself as a parent will damage the fundamentals of your relationship with your child, as it undermines the reciprocity you need to tune in to who they are.

I am sometimes guilty of this. When I get wedded to an image of myself as the perfect mum, it gets in the way of me *being* a mum. I go past good enough, looking for better, and end up exhausted, wired and resentful. In the past, I not only wanted to parent well, I wanted people to know I parented well. Now, the people I want to know I was a good parent are my own kids: as they grow into adulthood and away from me, I want the appreciation from them that they are evolutionarily programmed not to give. They are wired to question the status quo, to grow from the previous generation into something better. My teenage and young-adult kids do a wonderful piss-take of me: closed eyes, nodding head, pious and righteous – 'I sacrificed so much; I didn't go out for years; lay beside you in your bed; I was always there for you . . .' They scoff; I smart.

In the 'Good Enough' chapter, I introduced lots of peak-parenting positions – the healthy eaters, the activities junkies, the school-place seekers, the co-sleepers – and I gently questioned if rock-solid certainty of *any* extreme position was a helpful parenting strategy. But perhaps the most insidious peak-parenting position is that of the internet-perfect parent.

Getting stuck in your parenting image – be that your perfectly dressed baby, your yummy-mummy persona, your tidy, co-ordinated house or a particular ethos or ideology of parenting you are trying to keep to perfectly – will get in the way of being a good-enough, relationship-based parent. Perfectionism is an evil dictator: It gets very good press because, unfortunately, it is a very attractive dictator. We forget how evil it is as we are swayed by its superficial appearance. Perfectionism is fuel for depression, anxiety, eating disorders, obsessive-compulsive disorder – basically, for your own misery.

If perfectionism has been your master, now is always the time to change it; otherwise, it is also going to be a potential toxin in your kids' environment, interfering with your attachment with and your joy in them.[xxiii] Of course, it may also place relentless high expectations into their brains, too, and undermine their compassionate acceptance of themselves and of the imperfect here and now.[xxiv]

If perfectionism, and its favourite conspirator, anxiety, are poisoning your life, be honest with yourself, and do the work or get the help you need to pull your standards back to good enough. Then find your tribe of imperfect, kind, curious parent-friends, who can relax in your ordinariness, support and neither compete nor compare. Breathe, relax and try to enjoy.

PART 2: TODDLERS AND PRE-SCHOOLERS

2.1
Toddler Tantrums, Star Charts and All That Jazz

Just before we move on to toddlers, I want to pause and think about the mindset of babies, because I think that will help us understand why toddlers can be both so frustrated and frustrating. Developmental psychologists hypothesise that a baby has no understanding of the world separate to itself – they are egocentric and omnipotent, engrossed in their own experience and needs. Imagine that: not having any understanding of anything other than your own feelings. And, even better, imagine if all your needs and wishes were, on the whole, met. To the baby, in fact, it might seem as if they are in charge, controlling their parents. They feel hunger, they cry and are magically fed; they feel wet or dirty, they cry, and are cleaned and changed; they feel tired, and are put to sleep.

But all living things are wired to move towards independence. And so the baby starts to crawl and explore, and their wishes change from the quite simple (food, drink, sleep, comfort, being dry), to more complex (toys, standing up, wanting to copy others, sticking their fingers in a plug socket). They move from a position where what they wanted was allowed and generally met pretty promptly to having that thwarted, both by their own capacity and by the adults surrounding them. Through this, the toddler begins to recognise that others are separate, and, exploring with their own autonomy, they discover that the world is not as compliant to their wishes as it once seemed to be. In the toddler world that means a) exerting their right to put their own shoes on and b) not being able to put them on.

Therefore, as a parent, you have to move into managing more difficult behaviour – more wilful, more unpredictable, more irrational behaviour. And in so doing, you look for advice and wisdom. You find yourself in the supermarket with a small someone who has thrown themselves on the floor, hysterical, because they want to push the trolley *that they literally can't push,* or negotiating about why ballet pumps are not suitable footwear for the rain when you have a train to catch.

Surely parents have worked out the best way to manage this? Surely the psychologists and paediatricians can offer certainty about what is the best thing to do? I'm afraid not.

Over the last few generations, there have been rapid changes in beliefs and practices about disciplining children. Raising their five children just after the Second World War, my stylish and fun-loving grandparents were not wholly of the 'seen-and-not-heard' ethos, but also were not opposed to, on occasion, using a horse whip on their children's legs. My warm and funny parents had different ideas: raising their three children in the 1970s, although this was a time when schools were still allowed to use the cane, they thought the use of the whip was wrong. They would, however, slap the palms of our hands sometimes. When I came to parenting, after the turn of the millennium, the pendulum had swung away from any type of physical punishment at all, and I thought slapping was wrong. The zeitgeist of parenting was all about the behavioural school of psychology through Gina Ford and TV shows like *Supernanny*. The idea of 'time out' entered common parlance, and we were all about praising good behaviour with star charts and ignoring the bad. More recently, views have changed again, with time out seen as coercive and experts moving towards gentle or mindful parenting. This is a more child-focused approach, looking for the meaning behind their behaviour through understanding; and helping and supporting children to manage difficult or big emotions, rather than ignoring or punishing. But bringing this bang up to date, I also see a backlash against gentle parenting: that it is unsustainable for parents, requiring unrealistic levels of patience.

How do you find your way through these conflicting styles and theories? When discussing my limited success with behaviourism and sleep training, I ended up at a point of advocating firm and kind. This isn't something I made up. Parents have been shown to vary in two over-arching ways, and these are both on continuums. The first continuum, the one I sum up as 'kind', is actually a scale of how warm to cold parents are in their interactions with their children: warm parents are interested, engaged and positive, affectionate and loving, whilst cold parents are disengaged, unaffectionate, negative and unkind. The second continuum, the one I sum up as 'firm', runs from consistent, strict parenting with clear rules on one end to lax, boundary-less parenting on the other. These two continuums can be plotted against each other to create four 'types' of parenting, as on the diagram on the next page.

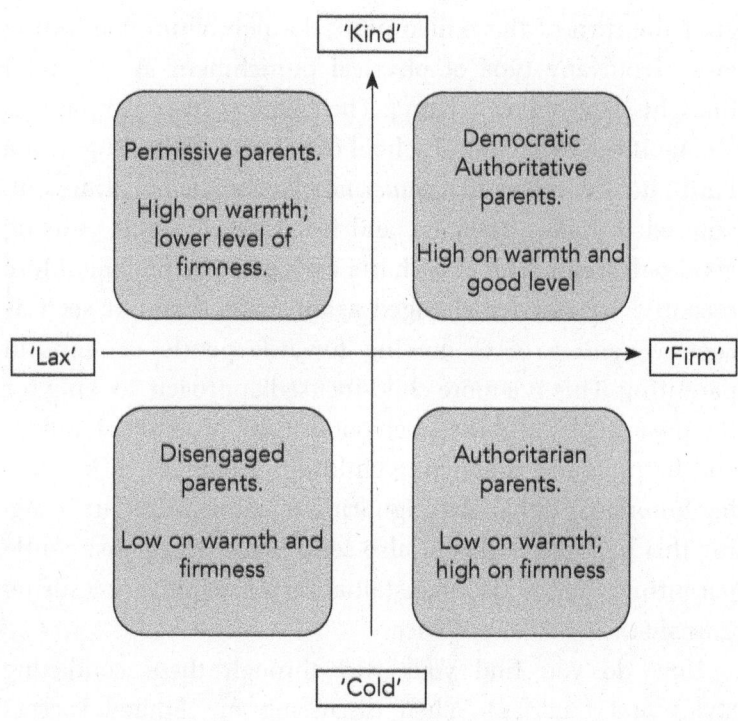

There is a remarkable consensus in the psychological research literature that the authoritative parent, who is firm and kind, is associated with better child outcomes. There is, however, perhaps a lack of agreement as to what firm and kind looks like in real life.

MY JOURNEY TO BECOMING A WORSE BEHAVIOURIST – PART II
Becoming a child clinical psychologist at the end of the twentieth century meant I had had a very deep schooling in the behaviourist theory and practice. Research shows that techniques such as reward charts and time out work, and blooming Supernanny was demonstrating them on national TV on a weekly basis. I was, at that time, a believer. Working in a psychiatric hospital

with children, we could have excellent results in turning children's behaviour around with these sorts of methods.

My doubts came later. And they were three-fold. Firstly, at work, I moved from the controlled environment of a hospital to work on Sure Start projects in a local deprived community.[11] Secondly, I had my own children. And then, thirdly, I returned to the research.

My doubts at work began when I found myself going into multi-problem families, dealing with their own mental- and physical-health problems, trauma, failure and poverty, armed with the inadequate tools of the behaviourist, such as praise, ignoring, stickers and rewards. I remember one family in particular. They were high service users; the mum had a learning difficulty and the dad had a criminal record. Neither of them worked. They were polite and nice when I visited – they offered me a cup of tea, they cleared a space on the sofa for me to sit down. They didn't turn the TV off. The house felt sparse – there was none of the normal (to my middle-class eye) clutter of family life: no pictures on the wall, no bookshelves, no framed photos. The toys were like the ones you see in a doctor's waiting room – slightly random, definitely broken and grubby and seemingly ill matched to the children. I was visiting at the behest of the nursery, as their eldest child was out of control. And he was. The parents felt defeated and uninterested, not only by their children, but also by my visit – one in a series from middle-class professionals trying to support them. Occasionally, the child went too far and he hurt himself, or his brother, or disturbed them, or broke one of their few possessions, and then they yelled at him or pulled him off.

---

11 Sure Start was a UK government initiative to improve the chances of young children in deprived localities.

Where was I to start with this as a psychologist in a one-hour weekly home visit? The health or education professionals see a family struggling to control their children and a psychologist is an obvious referral, but we don't have the sort of magic wand that can transform problems like these, which are built on multi-systemic issues. Getting through the day was hard work for these parents: organising food, getting their children dressed and trying to get them to nursery. Devoid of hope, with no job prospects and with little capacity to engender change in their own lives, their response to their son's misbehaviour was a classic projection of blame or responsibility: to label *him* as a problem.

I remember trying to explain the reformative power of praise and attention to this family, and how a star chart could be a useful tool to remember to provide praise. They said they'd give it a go. The next week, when I returned, they explained how their son had torn up the star chart after I left, and they'd given up. They hadn't shifted from the specific suggestion about star charts to the more general idea of praise, and so I tried to explain it again. I battled on over the weeks, trying to generate some change, but with little evidence that I had.

What I learnt working with families like this was that it was clearly difficult for them to keep alive the principle of increasing the good interactions with their child. I got this. It is hard to hold on to being kind or firm if your life is full of loss. But as a child-psychologist mum, in my calmer home and with better resources, I thought it could be different. At that point, I did believe I could train my child with my behavioural methods – and that I had the physical and mental means to do so. The positive stuff I found pretty easy: I enjoyed playing with my son, and we had a strong relationship; he was regularly praised, and we had a heap of good times, me and him. But he was a child who had a strong will and was often defiant. And he had a lot of temper tantrums when he didn't get his own way.

I remember his first tantrum well. Returning from the local shopping centre, my toddler initially just arched his back going into the car seat, reluctant and whiny. After gently wrestling him in, ten minutes later I stopped the car, as I thought he was having an epileptic fit. He was hysterical. As a psychologist, I was familiar with toddler tantrums (and, actually, epileptic fits), but this outburst in my own child, so small and previously delightful, meant that at first, I didn't realise what was going on.

However, I had been drilled on the importance of rewards and consequences, and I had experience of seeing them work in the psychiatric-hospital setting. It was almost like I had the behavioural psychologists on my shoulder, judging me. And so when my son didn't do as he was told, hit out or had temper tantrums, I thought I should do something. And the thing I thought I would do is be firm: he would always have the consequence of time out from whatever activity he was involved in, away from adult attention.[12]

Twenty years on, I'm not sure any of the time outs I did with him really worked. Of course, I don't have the benefit of a control with another identical child brought up by a less-firm-and-more-kind me to directly compare to, so I'll never actually know. Maybe if I hadn't done this, I'd have found that he dropped out of school and was on drugs by now, but my son is doing great. The time outs, when he sat on our bottom step with a timer, helped me feel as though I had a plan and a structure, and I liked feeling that I knew what I was doing. I often 'won' the battle: he stopped doing whatever it was or

---

12 Sorry, son – I was too firm. In my defence, I would also say I played hours of football with you in the park. In the rain. And I don't even like football.

received the message it was not acceptable. But his behaviour didn't change much in his childhood.

So, did I win the 'war'? I'm not sure I did in either the medium or the long term. In the medium term, he remained a defiant child and didn't really change his behaviour to avoid time out, as the theory and the books suggested he would. And in the longer term, I realised that he is fiercely independent and private and resents any interference (as he sees it)/intervention (as I see it) in his life from me as his mum. More than anything, he hates being told what to do. In my opinion, this is in his DNA. Time out didn't make it any better and may have made it worse; it didn't help him or teach him to manage this tendency in himself, he didn't calm down and it often made him cross, and so the situation would escalate. By the point he was in time out, I don't believe that my son cared two hoots what he was missing – by then his furious behaviour was driven by his own beliefs ('this isn't fair') and feelings (probably rage and indignation). And these thoughts and feelings, which the behaviourists ignore, were a far stronger influence than the loss of adult attention or not taking part in his activity.

I was an effective behaviourist in that I was for the most part consistent. I will always remember him saying to his little sister, 'There's no point in arguing, Mum never, ever changes her mind.' On one level, I felt proud; I knew how important consistency was in behaviour management. On another level, I felt perturbed. My son knew I was consistent and yet it hadn't made a blind bit of difference to his behaviour: he argued with me throughout his childhood about every last thing I told him to do. It may well be that I never, ever changed my mind, but he never, ever did as he was told. Did my consistency make any positive difference? Or did it exacerbate his natural defiance?

Would it have been better to teach by example, and show him what backing down or compromise look like? In retrospect, I think I not only sometimes sacrificed kind on the altar of firm, but also lost lots of opportunities to understand him, and to teach him about himself. Now he's all grown and quite, quite wonderful, I still think he could have benefited from understanding more about how changing your mind and admitting you've got things wrong are important. Maybe I should have taught him that by showing it?

Since those days, I have also dived deeper into the research, as I wanted to understand why what is meant to work didn't work for me. Firstly, it's always worth remembering when the clinicians say things like 'research has shown . . . time out works', they are always citing an average improvement, and rarely an improvement for everyone. But there are also holes in the time-out research, specifically in that it generally involves relatively short follow-up periods: say, a day, week, month. Research like this cannot give us long-term answers as to what sort of an adult the child will become because it simply does not run for that long. They don't say whether locking horns with my son made him more defiant or saved him from a delinquent future.

Also, this type of research has often been done in very different settings from a normal family home; for example, very controlled environments, like the psychiatric hospital I worked in myself, where a team of staff would be responding in a consistent way. When it is done in community settings, the research protocol tends to unlock an enormous amount of support and intervention for parents – much more than the once-weekly visit to struggling families I could offer as part of a normal community service.

So the research does not reflect the normal hurly burly of family life, where it is just not possible to be 100 per cent consistent and not change your mind; where it is difficult to notice every behaviour of your child and always follow through with praise or a consequence. Inevitably, you end up giving your child attention for the wrong thing and inadvertently 're-inforce' the behaviour you are trying to eliminate. I have come to believe that in real-life parenting, the aforementioned 'partial reinforcement schedule' (see p. 45) is unavoidable. That is, sometimes, you will have to unwittingly 'give in' to their wails or not praise something else because you are juggling with multiple demands.

But my final problem with the time-out research specifically is that a lot of it, that apparently 'shows' behaviour principles work, does so within an escalating situation of firmness that, imho, can easily tip into abusive. For example, from one study about what to do if a child comes out of time out it states: 'following initial escape the child was placed in an empty closet and prevented from leaving by blocking the door opening with plywood and spanking-enforced escape prevention (i.e. following initial escape the child was spanked on the buttocks with an open hand)'.[xxv] You'll be relieved to hear I didn't slap my son, nor place him in a closet blocking the exit. Is that why time out didn't work with him? These aren't things I want to do; they cross a line for me.

But even if you avoid slapping and closets, it is hard not to tip into too firm when you go down a behavioural route. Fundamentally, behaviourists believe that children should do what their parents tell them. But they never have and never will. Even when my mum and her siblings were hit with a horse whip, they didn't behave perfectly: they simply spent more time away from their parents wandering free, and also made sure that their bad behaviour was better hidden. Holding the belief that compliance is wholly achievable is bad for your blood pressure as well as your relationship with your children. I lost the opportunity to teach my son to calm down; instead, I went head to head in a battle of wills, underpinned by the belief that he should do as I say and that if I backed down, I'd lose my authority. Now, with twenty extra years as a mum and psychologist under my belt, I don't think you do lose your authority if you 'back down'; I think you demonstrate the compromise and flexibility that we desperately need to see in adult life. You show the change you want to be. And most of all, you protect your relationship with your child.

So my own experience at work and at home, with sleep training and with temper tantrums, has led me to believe that behaviourism hasn't got all the answers, particularly when behaviour is driven by strong emotion. I also now better understand how the research indicating that this works lacks application in real-life settings, and it goes to places that in my opinion are too harsh.

GENTLE PARENTING?

Gentle parenting, on the surface, would address these worries. It expands parents' focus from the behaviour of the child to considering the feelings and thinking behind it. Instead of seeing the answer to your child's tantrums as being in time out, it would have you ask, 'What is going on for them when they have a temper tantrum?' The gentle-parenting approach would be one where you hold the boundary ('No, you can't wear your ballet shoes in the rain'), but also name and acknowledge the feelings involved ('I know you feel really sad and upset about that; it's really hard. Ballet shoes are lovely, and it would be great to wear them, I understand, I get it.') Gentle parenting would then have you sit with and comfort the child whilst they calm down.

This is a good thing... in principle. It certainly mirrors the type of approaches I use in my therapy sessions with older children and adolescents: that is, I am looking at their thoughts and feelings, as well as their environment. Indeed, I see the psychology of anyone to be made up of five basic components. The first four are internal: their feelings, thoughts, behaviour and physiology (for example, their hormones and arousal levels). The final one is the context they are in. This includes the immediate environmental factors that the behaviourists look to for managing behaviour, such as your reaction to them, time out, etc., but also more distal elements, like sociocultural context, systemic deprivation and poverty. So when I work with people or families in clinic, I am using this sort of framework to help them understand themselves.

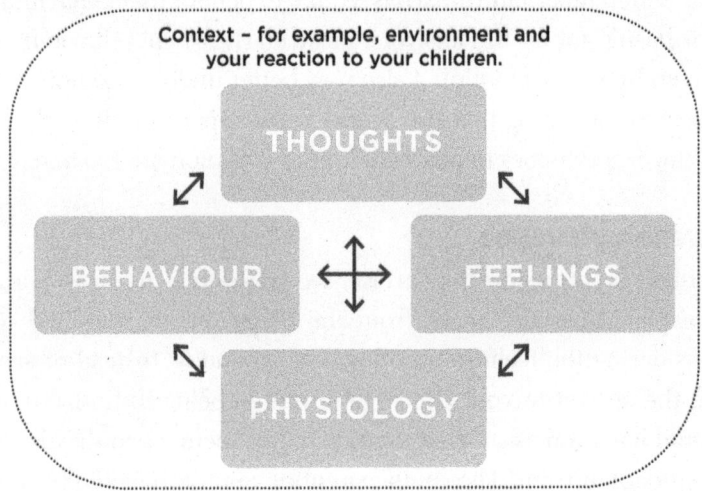

So my own experience of parenting and my disillusionment with the behavioural method and my clinical experience of working with children, and especially adolescents, might naturally lead me to a gentle-parenting position of helping them understand their thoughts and feelings. Children's behaviour is more complex than whether it is reinforced or not: when my son got upset, he stopped caring about my attention or whether he was joining in on the game and instead was driven wholly by the internal factors behaviourists ignore: his own thoughts and feelings. In addition, my manifesto aim of helping children to develop emotional competence in this incredibly changed, fast-paced world would also point towards gentle parenting. I constantly preach a philosophy of empathy and curiosity to parents to help them understand their older children. In retrospect, yes, I wish I had done more gentle parenting with my son. That I'd sat with his feelings more, held him more and been with him or explained his internal world more.

But I am not wholly convinced by the gentle parenting ethos, and that is for two reasons. The first is because I'm just not sure how feasible it is. And the second is that, like behaviourism, I think it can tip parenting into extreme, possibly perfectionistic aims.[13]

First of all, the feasibility aspect. Gentle parenting seems practically and emotionally difficult – to sit and wait with your toddler whilst they have a tantrum seems to preclude the fact that there may be other children, other work, somewhere to be or any time pressure. Gone is the bundling them in the car with the wrong shoes on and sorting it out when you get there. I own my privilege as a middle-class mum who worked part-time and had considerable resources to put into my parenting, but gentle parenting has a whiff of even more privilege to it. Time out may not achieve its medium-term aim of stopping the tempers or aiding compliance, but it does have the short-term advantage that you can get on and cook the fish fingers.

But also, I'm not sure I could have done it emotionally. Parenting babies and toddlers is a slog: it is a long lesson in giving up a whole heap of your own time, money, energy and yourself to care for someone else. I genuinely love being with babies and toddlers, and those years were some of the happiest of my life, but they were also the toughest. I was often

---

[13] A third reason is that there is very little research on gentle parenting. See Dr Ana Aznar from RecParenting at https://www.recparenting.com/for-parents/gentle-parenting-is-it-best/ for a summary.

exhausted, exasperated and frustrated. I'm not sure that I would have needed the expectation of myself to be more patient, kinder and constantly keep in mind my children's feelings – and I think about other people's feelings for a living! I'm good at intuitively picking up on others' feelings and motivations, and putting them into words, but I don't think I would have had the wherewithal to do that at times of high tension in such an active way, as well as get them fed, watered and out the door to nursery and school, with all the right stuff *and* get myself to work on time, too.

BEHAVIOURISM, GENTLE PARENTING, EXTREME PARENTING AND PERFECTIONISM

But secondly, I guess why I have reservations about both behaviourism and gentle parenting is because I'm not sure that *any* parenting strategy taken to the extreme is helpful. We are looking for the messy middle of good-enough relationship-based parenting here. Each of these ethoses intrinsically proposes that adherence to a model of parenting will improve the outcome by some marginal degrees, taking you away from parenting as yourself, or in a relationship. They can also contribute to a belief that your parenting is largely responsible for your child's outcome, every single thing you do matters: and therefore that you can never lose your shit.[14] That if your child has the archetypal meltdown in the supermarket, you need to be able (from the behavioural perspective) to give an immediate appropriate consequence or (from the gentle-parenting perspective) hear and understand their big emotions.

---

14 For a clarification on losing shit, I mean shouting, and not hitting. I do think you should attempt to go zero on a behaviour (hitting others) that is actually illegal between two adults. If you do end up hitting your child, I recommend a) apologising b) looking at ways you can get some more support/help/therapy in your life.

This is not to say I am an advocate of losing your shit, but I think holding the standard that you never do, or that you always react in accordance with your parenting ethos, will make it more likely that shit-will-be-lost – because that is what definitive standards and expectations do: they put pressure on a situation and make you uptight. As soon as you fail to be 100 per cent gentle, you feel like you've failed and berate yourself, or worse, blame your child for not responding to your gentle ways. Your child will not magically behave better because you have been mindful and thoughtful around your behaviour-management ethos. Thus, you will be constantly judging either yourself, or them, as not good enough. It takes you away from relationship-based parenting, as it takes you away from your own self.

You may even begin to dread parenting your child, as you can't reach your self-imposed standards derived from endless IG posts or well-meaning books. It's a warning sign if you find yourself wanting to spend less time with them because you are so worried about getting it right. You may feel your nemesis 'how-you-want-to-be-seen' self is taking over, rather than your true self. Perhaps you start looking for labels for your kid because, despite all your parenting efforts, they are still behaving badly: have they got ADHD? ASD? Dyspraxia? Sensory processing difficulties? Surely, it is not normal to behave like this? (Well, yes, it is: 91 per cent of three-year-olds have had a temper tantrum.[xxvi])

And whilst the research sets up the idea of a quadrant of firm and kind, my clinical experience has indicated to me that this isn't always just a case of more is better: as a parent, you can be *too* kind or *too* firm; and maybe the parenting pendulum has swung too far in both directions, into extreme parenting. That might look a bit like this:

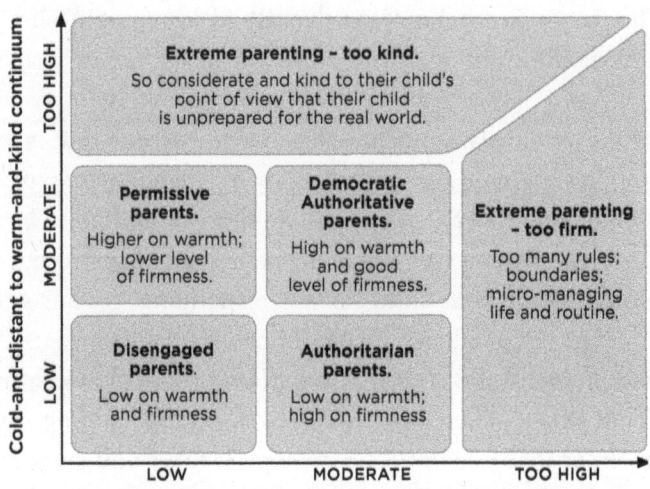

Behaviourism, as we have seen, can push a parent over the firm line, but even when it doesn't involve closets and planks of wood, I worry that we are starting children on an uber-analysed, constantly evaluated childhood: that we are giving them too much feedback on their behaviour. Star charts are no longer something a parent makes with a pen and paper, but are shiny, magnetic consumer items, with multiple spaces for tasks a pre-schooler should be doing each day! Yes, a star chart can be useful for teaching a toddler to use a potty, but do we really want to systematically observe and grade everything a child does each day and link it to a physical reward? There is some evidence that when we reward stuff that children actually like doing anyway, it makes them less likely to want to do it.[xxvii] But on a meta-level, does this contribute to the expectation in children that they should aim for perfection? Does it lead you to hold unrealistic aims for your children? Does it all contribute to a relentless hamster wheel of output or outcome?

Ultimately, I wonder if we are actually training kids to ignore their own thoughts and feelings and look to the opinions of others to judge their behaviour. I have concerns about this because so many of the young people I see in their teens or twenties are utterly possessed by the perceived opinions and approval of others. It's like a voice in their head querying their every word and action. Do they like me? Are they disappointed in me? Do they think I'm silly? How do they think I look?

And I'm not just talking about the defiant kids here, btw. I'm talking about the compliant ones, too. If you do have a very diligent, compliant child you might find that their star charts are training them as successfully as Pavlov's dogs into doing exactly what you want them to do. Training them into the pursuit of perfect behaviour, pleasing others and negating themselves. With behavioural interventions, we risk overlooking key parts of the manifesto – particularly emotional competence and building our relationship with them. We are indoctrinating them into a world where everything is graded: their behaviour, their fine and gross motor skills, their hobbies and interests, their academic ability and their appearance. And because there is always room for improvement, they never feel good enough.

The children and teenagers I see who seek the approval of others, at the expense of trusting their own opinions, well, they tend to be pretty miserable. They tend to make the wrong decisions: studying too hard chasing the good opinion of their teachers, choosing a university or course for status, rather than one they would enjoy, and complying with sexual demands of others, fearing their disapproval.

Yet, at the other extreme, with gentle parenting, are we training them to be self-indulgent, believing that the world revolves around their thoughts and feelings? Giving them an unrealistic expectation about how much other people will care? As a parent and a psychologist, I've seen too many kids who have kind, understanding parents and never any sanctions whacking other kids over the head with a toy train at three years old, or taking ket at fifteen. The gentle-parenting proponents would say I am misrepresenting them here, and that it can still have boundaries. I'm sure that's right, but my concern is that we may be raising kids to be what I call 'pretty and precious', believing not only that their feelings are always valid (and they are not), but also that someone else needs to change their behaviour on account of them.[15]

So instead, I'm drawn to the messy middle of parenting, where you accept the limits you have on being able to control either their short-term behaviour or their long-term outcome. You are not in control of this. Yes, give your toddler some consequences, especially if their behaviour impacts others (for example, hitting), but don't expect them to not act like a toddler, until, well, they are not a toddler. Because mostly, they grow out of these behaviours. Yes, try to acknowledge and understand their feelings, but you don't need to always stop what you are doing to do so: they have got big feelings, and they need help to begin to understand these, but I would argue that it's probably unhelpful to always have their feelings dominate family life. Their feelings are important, but so are other things.

I would look at the risks of getting stuck in any one ethos or dogma, in that it puts expectations on you and your family that can backfire. I'm saying be firmish and kind. And I would remind you that you are allowed to get this wrong. You only

---

15 An unpopular view, I fear, that feelings are not always valid. Feelings are often based on untrue narratives in our heads. Sometimes feelings are literally madness. I feel that a misunderstanding has arisen in the meaning of 'validating feelings' between accepting that someone feels like that and that they need understanding and empathising with, which is always important, and accepting that their feelings are based on reality and truth, which is often not therapeutically helpful.

need to be good enough on firmish and kind. That is why I say good enough is the greatest of the three principles.

In conclusion, I want to say two things. Firstly, what my experience reminded me is that the most important behavioural tip is to set a good example. In the psychology literature, this is called behavioural observation: your kids will learn by watching you. So show up; don't hold an ideology so tightly that you don't actually want to be with them because it's too hard to reach your own standard. Let go of the expectation that they will always comply or behave. It's normal for them to experiment and be, at times, more concerned with their own wishes in the moment than your opinion. Yes, teach them that behaviour has consequences, but don't shame them for behaving in a way that is completely normal at that age. Be kind: de-escalate, distract, use humour. Try to manage your own feelings to put something positive in the space between you and your kids, but be compassionate to yourself when you don't. Here again, you will be teaching by example – you are human; you get it wrong – so just apologise and take ownership of your feelings. This is a good-enough way to be.

The second thing is this: have fun. Surely parenting at the beginning of the twenty-first century, with all our mod cons and freedoms, should mean that we enjoy our kids? And through that enjoyment build the relationship that underpins all behaviour management. A huge chunk of what I learnt about behaviour management is in the next chapter: play. And on this, the gentle-parenting gurus and the behavioural researchers all agree – that the research shows time out only works in the context of increased positive interaction between parent and child. Why? Because kids are a no-credit bank: you need money in the bank to spend money. You will need a good relationship in the bank and lots of positive interactions to gain compliance. You need to put in the hours with the Lego and the doll's house.

2.2
Play and Joy

I finished the last chapter extolling the benefits of play as a behaviour-management tool, as a sweetener to tempt you in. I could have instead reeled you in with a discussion of the importance of play to the learning agenda, perhaps calling the chapter 'Play to Get Ahead' or something like that. And both of these are true: I can firmly report that playing with your child, in the ways we will discuss, will improve behaviour, and will also maximise learning opportunities. It's just that I don't think they are the most important factors in the argument for play. Indeed, I think focusing on these, and perhaps learning in particular, can strip play of its joyful benefits. So I'm putting a bid in for play for manifesto reasons. I'm proposing prioritising two approaches: for you to engage in child-led play as the starting point for building a reciprocal relationship with your child; then them having lots of opportunities for free play as they get older without adult intervention, as the foundations of joy and happiness.

Play seems to be an innate and biological urge, wired into not only us, as humans, but young mammals, too. It is a feature of every society, throughout time, and, as such, has piqued the interest of anthropologists, sociologists and psychologists.

Why do children play? We've studied the hell out of it, analysed its purpose and nature, and possibly, in doing so, we have inadvertently been a factor in its downfall. Because any Joe Bloggs on the Clapham omnibus can tell you the purpose of play. They could tell you about an early-years agenda, and how play is important for kids' socialisation and learning. They could even possibly tell you that play is important for a child's sense of identity, and for cognitive, emotional and physical development. For their hand–eye co-ordination. But in such a comprehensive analysis of play we have perhaps contributed to the destruction of the thing that we were studying. A bit like all the tourists swarming to Venice or the Galapagos Islands. In our rush to witness and celebrate, we inadvertently annihilate.

In Chapter 1.2, we saw how the first step in relationship-based parenting is the baby–parent attachment. I suggested that key to attachment is the one-to-one interaction of you showing up a lot and responding to your baby's cues. I made an analogy between attachment and dancing with your baby, mostly in your arms, face-to-face, jigging together in synchronicity. In the Still Face Experiment on p. 36, we saw an example of the goo-goo-gah-gah parenting, and this kind of baby talk seems to be a universal phenomenon – a natural thing most of us do when faced with a baby. We mostly, it seems, speak baby. So I'm going to put the case to you for play as the second step of relationship-based parenting, but I think this is a less natural one for many parents. Sadly, we adults often seem to have forgotten the language of play. We had it once, when we were children, presumably, but we have had it socialised out of us. Perhaps because, at some point, we were compelled to work hard, get on, be serious and be in control; or perhaps because we are hijacked by the learning agenda as parents. Either way, many of us seem to lose our playfulness.

And this, I think, is a shame, because in relationship-based parenting you are trying to respond reciprocally to your toddler, and your toddler speaks play. They are beginning to learn normal language, but it will be years before they can clearly tell you what is going on in their mind, and their language skills are nowhere near expressive enough yet. For your relationship to continue to grow and develop with them, you have to meet them where they are, and where they are is, of course, playing.

Going back to my attachment dancing analogy again, in the toddler years they are no longer in your arms, but dancing near you, and wanting your attention. They will want you to hold their hand, or to do that thing when they stand on your feet whilst you dance, consequently dancing with you, in synchrony. They want you to respond to their moves and twirl them around. Sometimes they will go off for a bit and dance with their friends, but they will want to know where you are, and to come back to you. What they won't want is to be ignored; nor will they want every dance you have together to actually be a lesson where they have to learn new steps or dance in some particular way.

The responsibility for making your relationship with your child work falls primarily on you, the adult, but it has to adapt to what your child is giving off as a separate, unique human. A good-enough parent takes that responsibility seriously, but that doesn't mean they have to control, structure or organise it. Crucially, they let their child also shape the relationship; they respond to what their child is bringing, they 'read the room', they get to know the child in front of them. It's about responding to the kid you've got, rather than parenting from a script or to fulfil your own needs.

When I think of the relationship difficulties I see in my clinical work, they often occur when reciprocity fails, and frequently mean the parent is not really seeing and hearing their child where they are. There are different reasons why that might be. As we saw in the toddler tantrum chapter, parents sometimes view the parental relationship as one of control, and of imposing their will and way of doing things on to the child. Or they might see what they want to see, rather than the child they've got, and perhaps even be a little too kind. Or they might have their eyes so firmly on the highest potential of the child that they don't see the stress that working to that creates. Often, even the most attentive parents don't really see their child at the stage of life they are at, and try to keep them younger or hurry them older.

In the toddler years, when language is not fully developed, play is how a child communicates. So, child-led play lets you get to know the child you've got. It allows you to start to sit and listen, not necessarily to what they are saying, but what they are showing, and it trains you to meet them where they are, rather than where you want them to be. A crucial skill for every parent, I think.

CHILD-LED PLAY

My introduction to child-led play was when I worked as a clinical psychologist in Sure Start. As part of that, I led Webster-Stratton Incredible Years parenting groups in local community centres.[16] I don't remember exactly, but I expect I may have used the very sweeteners I outlined at the start of the chapter to encourage attendance at a weekly parenting group in a deprived area of London. That is, we attracted parents with the promise of behaviour management for toddlers, or possibly maximising the potential of their child. And, whilst it may seem

---

16 These parenting groups are a community intervention to give parents skills to manage their young children, focusing on play, praise, effective limit setting and handling misbehaviour.

at odds with these aims, the first two sessions were taken up with child-led play.

What do I mean by child-led play? I mean sitting with your toddler or young child and being with them whilst they play. I mean following their lead and providing an engaged but not dominating audience. And I mean not structuring or organising their play – just showing an interest but not taking over. So make yourself a cup of tea, get on the floor and play what they are playing. It sounds simple, yet most adults find this really hard.[17]

I touched on the reasons why adults find it difficult above, but let's just think about this a bit more. I think some adults find it easier than others to give themselves over to play – grandparents, for example, or childless godparents or aunts and uncles. But as parents, we have such a strong narrative of having to be in control. Why? Do we fear the little buggers will take over if we give up the reins of control for ten minutes: that it might get a bit *Lord of the Flies*? Do we fear that if we let our guard down, we will lose our authority, show our vulnerability, they will take advantage? We have been socialised into the 'do-better-and-get more' society, where playing with them at all can feel boring or a waste, when we could be teaching them something to 'get on' or 'get ahead' in life. Perhaps this is why play has been hijacked by the learning agenda: flick through any toy catalogue and you will see the language of industry and achievement: educational, learning, early years, development. So when we *do* play, we want to teach them that the oven and table go in the kitchen of the doll's house or that the Lego car should have one, two, three, four wheels. We pride ourselves on the little bits of learning we can shoehorn in.

---

17 For more advice on how to play Webster-Stratton's book (1992). *The Incredible Years: A Trouble-shooting guide for Parents and Children aged 3–8*.

And learning is, of course, important, but what I'm saying is you are allowed to forget it, and just sit and be with your child's play: ask *them* where they want you to put the oven. Maybe they want you to balance it on your nose. And see that this car they have made has five wheels, without giving a lecture on how that would not really work because wheels all need to face the same direction, or feeling you always need to count in that laborious, slightly pompous, self-righteous way parents do to teach. I suspect your kid will get counting; you don't need to get them doing it earlier or quicker. That doesn't fast-track them to academic success. If you are not sure what to do, giving a slow, gentle running commentary on their play is a good way of paying attention and showing interest. Like the commentary of a cricket match rather than Formula One. Train yourself, when they are a toddler, to be with them, where they are, watching and listening to what they bring.

Of course, there is *an* agenda here. The agenda is to get to know your kid and to open up the channels of communication that you are going to need so much in later years. You are at once deepening your relationship with them and, through their experience of being seen and heard, laying down a foundation for them of how to be with others. When you let a child lead play you have to let go of your control, your desire to do things 'right' and your drive for improvement; you are teaching them instead about being in the moment, not moving forwards, and you will see the benefits of this downstream in childhood and adolescence.

For many parents it feels so unnatural: *we* weren't played with like this; it did *us* no harm! Perhaps, or perhaps not. But isn't it what we all want in life? Someone to stop with the busyness and pull up to us with an open heart and hear what is going on in our minds? I don't know whether it was done in the past – I am not a historian. Maybe in the past it was all about the patriarchal hierarchy. But I can only say that now, in this fast-paced, emotionally complex world, a reciprocal relationship with your child, I think, gives them the best foundation for my manifesto aims.

When I ran parenting groups, I and my other group leaders would extol the benefits of play for a couple of hours and encourage parents to try it before the next week's session. Usually, only one or two did, but then they did our work for us: they were evangelical on the benefits of play. They came back with tales of reformed behaviour and increased compliance. Sometimes they loved the play themselves, and sometimes they hated it, but they all recognised the benefits. Later in the group programme, we did focus more directly on behaviour management, such as time out and consequences. But genuinely, I do not remember anyone coming back evangelical about these. It was the play that the parents found transformational.

And whilst my observations from running groups are not a scientific study, it is worth repeating that, as far as I can tell from the research, *all* the successful strategies for improving behaviour, be they from the hardline behaviourists or the gentle-parenting proponents, would have it that spending positive time in play with your toddler is the first step in improving behaviour. This point of agreement often gets missed when the culture wars break out between different parenting experts.

The discipline message is so appealing to us, it's so easy to get drawn back in. I remember a mum returning to me a year or so after she had attended one of the groups. Over time, her child's behaviour had worsened again, and she wanted to see me for a top-up. As we chatted, and I heard how naughty her child was being, I was drawn in to doubling down on the consequences for their behaviour. She paused, and said, 'Actually, I don't think that is what I need to do. Talking to you now, I realise I've forgotten to keep playing. That's what made the most difference from the group – when I started the playing.' I checked myself with a little bit of shame that *I'd* forgotten, too: it's so instinctive to try to control through the more forceful elements. Like the fable of whether the wind blows off a coat, or the sun shines it off: go sun, I say. If you can, Team Sun: shine your parenting warmth on the good stuff.

One more thing. As parents, there's always the temptation to get the chores done before we play. To use play as the prize for compliance: get dressed, eat your breakfast, wash your hands, tidy up the kitchen and then we'll play. In doing this, we risk making everything transactional. But children are poor at delayed gratification and will whinge and whine through the chores. My experience is that after they have had their time of one-to-one playing, they will be more amenable to instructions: giving them that time where they are in charge calms them. It's like you have credit in the parenting bank that they will then let you spend. Parents also often fear that when they start to play, they will be stuck there all day; but in fact, once engaged in child-led play, kids generally let you go or slip off and continue with the game themselves. But even if your child does protest when you leave, you will likely feel OK about setting that boundary – that you need to go now – because you know you have done your bit and won't feel guilty. You have passed the good-enough bar, and you get to go do the washing up/do your work/smoke a fag/whatever you want or need to do.

FREE PLAY

Another reason you can feel cool and comfortable walking away from child-led play is because this free play, either by themselves or side by side with others, is key, too. Indeed, whilst you know I don't think 'learning' is the most important thing about child-led play, you are actually teaching them up with the skills that will be necessary for free play: reciprocity, turn-taking and sharing of ideas. Remember toddlers are developing from the baby-position where they are the centre of the world, and everyone else is a character in their story. They don't have a theory of mind: they don't understand that other people are thinking and feeling things just as much as themselves. To play successfully with each other, children need to be able to take the point of view of their friend, co-create an imaginary game together, like a little thought bubble they are both contributing to. These skills take time to learn, and often need adults to scaffold the play whilst they do so. By scaffold, I mean be near by, lightly supervising, and offering occasional guidance to help keep them on track.

I was talking about the sharing of ideas in the paragraph above, but whilst we are on the subject of sharing, here's a little word on the sharing of belongings. Of course, to play successfully, some degree of sharing belongings is necessary, and kids need to understand that. But we, as adults, get a bit obsessed with this, like it is the most important thing we have to teach them – that it is a major personality flaw not to give up something we want because someone else wants it. Sharing belongings isn't really a huge part of adult life: I don't let my friends come to my house and rifle through my belongings, pick out their favourites and let them have them for a bit. I think when we parents get a bit stuck on the 'share-nicely' narrative, it is because our frenemy how-we-want-to-be-seen has shown up. We are playing the role of a good parent. What we are really trying to do when we insist on sharing is a misguided attempt to make children see someone else's point of view – the skill of empathy. But verbalising the dilemma teaches this more successfully than forcing them to surrender Thomas the Tank Engine to their friend. 'You both want the toy: that's really hard. What should we do?' might be the way to go. We don't need to force learning; we just need to plant the seed.

The purpose of the scaffolding when they are younger is that as they get older, we can withdraw our supervision and allow the adventure and joy of free play. But play has not only been hijacked by the learning agenda – it has become commodified and commercialised, and businesses have taken it over to squeeze every single bit of money they can out of it. They sell to parents' hopes and fears, to them wanting to be the best parent they can possibly be, seeking 'better' play opportunities for their children. So children no longer play in their homes and gardens – they play in huge warehouses, filled with plastic climbing materials. They follow 100-page booklets to make Lego sets that sit on a shelf, rather than having a dirty great box of old bits of Lego to build wondrous creations. Later on, they don't ride their bikes around the streets; instead, they do extreme BMX freecycling in designated skate parks. They don't so much go to the park with a ball but play FIFA on the PS5.

The changes in play over the last generations take it away from some of the fundamental things we know to be important about happiness. For example, we know in mental health that having an internal locus of control (a belief in our own agency and capability over ourselves) is key to mental wellbeing. Renowned psychologist and researcher Peter Gray argues that free play gives children an internal locus of control – a belief that what they do makes a difference – and that this protects them from anxiety and depression later in life.[xxviii] When we supervise and micro-manage children's play, they look and come to us to control, and do not discover their own power and capacity.

Many older children have now lost the opportunity for free independent play. A time that was traditionally under children's own control is now under the control of adults. Of course, there may be advantages to this, as sanitised environments, subject to health-and-safety measures, will be safer, and adult supervision may mean that unkindness or bullying won't go unchecked. Things weren't perfect when children had freedom to play.

The commodification of play undermines another root of happiness: acceptance of a good-enough present, and not in the always-wanting-more in the future. The business model of the play industry is in direct opposition to this, instead depending on creating dissatisfaction in kids with what they already have. That is the purpose of all those movie tie-in toys, of collect-the-set football cards and of in-game purchases. The hedonic principle means that kids quickly habituate to any new toy they get; it becomes the norm, and then they want more. They are sold more and more with the belief that better is just ahead, rather than good enough being here now. We indoctrinate into children the desire for new, faster, improved toys and games.

In the mental-health clinics, we have seen an increase of two different sets of kids: boys showing up at six, seven or eight for ADHD referrals and teenage girls with eating disorders and anxiety. We will come to both these groups again – in the childhood-education chapter for the boys, and in the 'Good Enough' and 'Holding On' adolescent chapters. For now, both, I think, could benefit from more play.

The boys can't sit still in their classrooms; they are full of energy and fidgety. Literally thousands of them every year are being diagnosed as 'having' ADHD, given a potentially lifelong diagnosis and often the corresponding medication. When I sat in CAMHS referral meetings, I used to find the swathes of referrals from Year 1 and 2 depressing.[18] Many of these boys were doing OK, until it was found that they could not meet an arbitrary societal requirement – that they sit still at a desk with a pencil in their hand. Other countries in the world do not demand this, and there is no evidence that an early ability to do it results in better long-term achievement. As I sat in the CAMHS meetings, listening to referral after referral, I found myself wondering how many of them would have been made and how many of these boys would be labelled, if there wasn't a requirement for them to sit still for so long each day? How would they be if left to free play? Were we labelling and medicating them into compliance? Maybe they didn't have ADHD; maybe they had insufficient-freedom disorder?

As for the second group – the girls striving for perfection, weighed down by the oughts, shoulds and musts of life – these girls, by their teenage years, have been socialised into believing that there is a right way, a neat way, to do things, and they've lost their playfulness, the joy of unpredictable fun, which involves embracing not knowing and chaos. Instead, weaned on keeping the rules, they end up constantly comparing, scared of putting a foot wrong and believing that nothing they do is good enough. Left to their own devices in play, they may have lined things up and made them neat, as girls often do place an in-built straitjacket on their own behaviour – but has adult-structured, commercialised play exacerbated that tendency, rather than loosened it?

---

18 CAMHS is the Child and Adolescent Mental Health Services, which is the NHS mental-health service for under-eighteens. Years 1 and 2 start at ages five and six respectively.

So I'm putting in a bid for the relationship-based parent to prioritise two different types of play at this age *and* going forward: first, particularly when children are very little, for you to listen and attend to them through child-led play; and second, as they grow, to gently tend their play, and then give them freedom to roam and play without you. In the move between these two types of play, you are beginning to traverse the ground between your attachment relationship with them and their relationships with other people. Both types mean, to some degree, giving up the parental control and trusting in the good-enough project.

But finally, I don't want you to forget one more thing about play – perhaps the most important thing of all. And that is joy. The fun of being silly together, of making do, of sharing a moment. For – and excuse me if I get a bit philosophical right now – what is a life without joy? Forget about establishing learning, growth and development in your child, for surely what we want more than anything for our kids now, and in their adult lives, is a sense of joy? A sense of playfulness, mischievousness and fun that they can take through to adulthood, and which will sustain them through the inevitable tougher times.

2.3
Good-Enough Food and Eating

Recent headlines about food and eating suggest that this is one area where we, society, are not meeting the good-enough bar. We know that rates of obesity and, conversely, eating disorders have sky-rocketed over the last generation.[xxix] So some kids are eating way too much, and some are eating way too little, and what I think is important to understand is these are two sides of the same coin; the problems are inextricably linked. There is a multi-dimensional problem, starting with societal issues, such as fundamental changes in the availability of food and the way we eat, often mediated by how we educate and parent around it, and ending with the most individualised stuff: the hunger, satiety and preferences of your own child.

In thinking about food and eating, we often hear from the dietitians and nutritionists about what is or is not healthy; we hear from the dentists about what is good for teeth; we hear from the fitness gurus and dieters about how to keep the body slim and beautiful, the latter often hiding their dieting advice in the more acceptable guise of health. Where are the psychologists in this? What do *we* know about how to raise a child to have a psychologically healthy relationship with food?

My definition of psychologically healthy eating comes from a wonderful book called *If Not Dieting, Then What?* by Rick Kausman. It involves two key components: intuition and nutrition.[xxx] Intuition means being able to listen to your body: what it fancies and what will satisfy you; and nutrition is being able to do this with a quantity and the types of food that keep you in reasonable health. Maintaining a balance between these two factors is, to me, psychologically healthy eating: good-enough eating.

The question for this chapter, then, is how to raise a child to do that, as you wean your baby, and then establish an eating pattern for your toddler and, moving forwards, your child and adolescent? How do you maximise the chances that they will eat joyfully with satiety and health in mind? To answer this question, we will need to return to our good-enough continuum; but before that, I think we need to consider this time of excess and the impact it has on our attempts to raise psychologically healthy eaters.

FOOD AND EATING IN THE CURRENT CONTEXT

In Chapter 2.1 on toddler tantrums, I described how in psychology there are five key factors we need to consider: four internal to us – feelings, thoughts, behaviour and physiology; and one external, which is the context. To help your child achieve psychologically healthy eating, you'll need to consider all five, but let's start by acknowledging the huge impact of social context on our eating and relationship to food.

A generation ago, when I started secondary school, we were told by the headteacher not to eat in our school uniform in the street, as this was thought to show the school in a bad light. In my local town, we didn't have McDonald's or any pizza restaurants. We barely ate out at all as a middle-class family: maybe once a year at a pub. The only takeaway food we ate was fish and chips.

We ate a roast on Sundays, and then the leftovers from that on Mondays and Tuesdays. Most of our food was freshly prepared by my mum, who had a part-time job but would have called herself a housewife. We ate round a table, together. We never had ready-made meals – did they even exist? We did, however, have many things that would now be considered unhealthy: pudding most days, homemade cake generally available, Angel Delight, sausages . . .

I tell you this because I think it illustrates the rapid societal changes that have contributed to the complexity of raising psychologically healthy eaters. We are raising our kids in times of unprecedented availability of convenient, cheap, delicious food. Our evolutionary history has prepared humans to eat more than we need in times of plenty to help us through the next interruption in our food supply, which now, for many of us, never comes. In addition, social conventions about when and where we are allowed to eat have been dropped. The pace of life has quickened – working parents do not have time to be making Cornish pasties from a leftover Sunday roast as my mum did. Fast food is pushed, marketed and widely available. To provide nutritionally rich, fresh food is expensive, complex and time-consuming. Largely, these societal changes have directed us towards consuming more ultra-processed foods, and often overeating.

But food availability and attitudes are not the only things to have changed over the last generation; there have also been massive changes in an appearance-driven culture. Whilst the glorification of thin started earlier, the last twenty years have seen a huge growth in mass and social media, which have led to us viewing an explosion of images and videos every day, most of which reinforce traditional images of slimness and attractiveness. We know that the more we view these images, the worse our body dissatisfaction, something we will be returning to later when we think about social media.[xxxi]

The changes in the food environment alongside body-image pressure has allowed the dieting industry to flourish. It's an industry that didn't exist seventy years ago, but which is now worth hundreds of billions of pounds. A business model that cleverly survives on its own failure to succeed, providing itself with an endless stream of return customers.[xxxii] A multi-billion-pound industry has been created in selling us (eating) less.

So we are raising our children to eat in a society that pinballs back and forth between at least three separate, often contradictory messages: those around food and eating; those around dieting and health; and finally, those around the way we are expected to look. I always think Sunday newspaper magazines are a perfect place to view these conflicting expectations. Over just a few pages, it is all laid bare. There are the pages encouraging us to eat: delicious recipes, often with high sugar and fat content; restaurant reviews; food advertisements (often for processed foods). Then, there are pages showing very thin, highly glamorous models or toned and slim celebrities. And finally, there are the pages with the latest fad diets or fitness crazes – these are ever changing, each one extolling the benefits or evils of different foods or a different method. The magazines represent a microcosm of attitudes in society: eat well and a lot, but be thin and glamorous , and stay healthy by not eating this or that. I sometimes wonder if we have gaslit ourselves into food/eating/weight/shape madness?

How do we change this for the next generation? How do we find a psychological and physical balance in these times of excess, contradiction and extremes? Our task in raising children to be psychologically healthy eaters is, I think, a unique one in the arc of history.

WHERE IS GOOD ENOUGH ON CHILDREN'S FOOD AND EATING?

In the first chapter, I introduced my good-enough continuum, with abusive on one side and perfect on the other, and most of us muddling along in the messy middle of good enough. How does that play out with food and eating? What is good enough here?

I'm pretty sure that it's uncontroversial to say that deliberately not giving a child enough to eat would constitute abuse. But is it abusive or neglectful to give your kid too much, or the wrong sorts of foods, so they end up overweight or obese? There has been much debate on this matter, but I don't think so.[xxxiii] Overeating reflects parents are too tired, too confused or possibly too poor to do any different. Cheap, quick food is often fattening food. Parents feeding children like this are usually eating like this themselves, perhaps relying too much on intuition in their food choices. I would also be respectful of the 'Health at Every Size' lobby who would argue that the health disadvantages of being overweight are overstated and often an effect of health inequalities or stigma. Yet raising a child on a high-sugar, high-fat, high-processed-food diet without an awareness of nutrition, or the capacity to choose it, is likely to lead them to a lifetime of being in a larger body, and whatever health complications that involves, as well as prejudice. I don't think any parent would choose this for their future child as they move to wean them. It may not be abusive, but it is probably less than good enough.

The risks of overeating and the obesity crisis in the Western world are well documented, but what of the other end of the good-enough continuum? Well, I believe there are also risks in providing a 'perfect' environment for food and eating for your child – and one of these is that you are not preparing them for the sociocultural environment they live in. When you are weaning them, sure, it's tempting to keep them in a little bubble of your food choices, but as they grow you have to prepare them for a world that has delicious food on nearly every corner. If your weaning or child-feeding environment just focuses on one dimension of food – health – you ignore, at your peril, the complex bio-psycho-social reasons why we eat. You risk overlooking the cultural, religious or historical meaning of food: how what we eat connects us to our communities, our heritage. You risk squashing out all the social pleasure around food – eating to celebrate or eating to connect: the shared sweets on the bus, the birthday cake – taking all the joy out of it through a ubiquitous health message. Food can become imbued with a moral judgment of being 'good' and 'bad', equating to 'healthy' and 'unhealthy'. And, most importantly, you don't teach your child – by example or their own experience – how to eat with moderation in plentiful supply, balancing intuition and nutrition.

Parents who try to provide a perfect, 'healthy' food environment for their offspring do it, of course, with love. They have perhaps reached child-rearing age having gone through their own journey with food, health, weight and shape. They may have had to learn the hard lesson that we need less food as we age. They have found a schedule of food and exercise that works for them, but that sometimes views food through the primary prism of health. They want their child to know what they have learnt from their experience, and so don't allow them to have that experience themselves and find their own way. They do it by providing a controlling environment for their child – an uber-'healthy' environment: a restrictive environment.

It's probably no surprise that in adults restrictive eating patterns, aka dieting, are linked to future eating disorders. What may be more of a surprise is that restrictive eating is linked to future overeating and to obesity, both through binge eating and through successive failed dieting attempts, leading to a slow ratcheting up of weight.[xxxiv, xxxv] Whilst this is not evidence that raising children in this way leads to these problems, a restrictive food environment does not prepare them for the society they will live in.

Let's think about how that can backfire: a child is raised in a home where there are a lot of restrictive practices – for example, not seeing on a day-to-day basis food with sugar or much fat, or increasingly no carbs, too, and receiving the messages that foods are 'healthy/good' or 'unhealthy/bad'. What do they do later? If they've mainly had rice cakes or apples for a snack, what do they do when they go to a birthday party on their own at six or seven, or when they go to a tween sleepover or they're on their gap-year travels at eighteen and have access to plentiful sweets, crisps and chocolates, or everyone around them is eating burgers or pizza? This creates an internal dilemma for the child: they know these foods are 'bad', but everyone else is eating them.

Well, there are a few ways out for them. Some of them might continue to restrict – they will create distance between themselves and their peers. For thousands of years food has been used to share and connect people, but our preoccupation with 'health' undermines this. Food perfection, and indeed all types of perfection, are linked with social disconnection.[xxxvi] The girl not eating the chips (and yes, it sadly often is the girl) will be noticed by all the other girls for sure, and that will likely create a disconnect between her and them. Or perhaps the more rebellious will eat the very thing they've been indoctrinated against, whether they want it or not, just because they can. They will likely struggle to stop eating when they are full, or when it stops being pleasurable, as, if food is not usually available, we tend to eat to excess on the rare occasions it is. Some of these 'overeaters' may then feel guilty and try to make amends by eating less the next day, or, even worse, through self-induced vomiting, laxatives or eating-induced-exercise. And in these three positions we have the possible roots of the different disordered eating patterns: anorexia, obesity and bulimia. What I think will be harder for them to do after being raised in a restrictive environment is to listen to their own bodies (intuition – I want some) and their own knowledge (nutrition – and now I've had enough).

But the risks go beyond just food and eating: they are the risks of exerting excessive control over our children, and not responding to who they are. We risk negating their individuality.

INTERNAL AND PSYCHOLOGICAL DRIVERS TO EAT

Full confession: I fell for the perfect-eating myth for a while when weaning my firstborn. At that time, there was one baby-feeding guru: Annabel Karmel. She had several books and a media presence and was all about preparing all your baby's food from scratch, in a particular order with a wide range of flavours presented. It made intuitive sense to me that if I gave my baby all these different flavours, they would develop a taste for them and not be fussy in the future. So I stayed up late at night, puréeing and mashing exotic vegetables for the next week's meals and freezing them in ice-cube trays. He ate everything, and at his first birthday had never had a single sweet. And I was wonderfully smug in my perfect mothering.

I was saved from my perfection by my son's free will and returning to work with less time to purée and mash. And whilst I'd hoped all that prep was going to give him a broad and wide palate for food, after his first birthday, he instead tried to refuse all fruit and vegetables until he was sixteen. Not wedded to a healthy-eating philosophy, I adapted and had to find a balance between what I wanted him to eat (the important nutrients that fruit and veg provide) and what he wanted to eat (white carbs and meat). When he was at nursery school, he had a daily piece of fruit, but we never expanded his repertoire beyond raisins and apples. I had be 'firm' to get him to eat a piece of vegetable at dinner, and under daily protest he did. And he continued to protest about that until he was sixteen. We all remember well sitting around the dinner table waiting for him to eat his broccoli with one of his friends when they were sixteen: eventually, the friend, leant across the table, pierced the broccoli with a fork and put it in his mouth. 'Come on, mate,' he said. 'We want to go.'

You see, expecting your child to eat in line with your ideas about perfect health ignores one other very important factor: that they are an individual with their own preferences, with their own internal drivers for eating and with their own tastes, and hunger and sense of satiety. You may have a child who fills up really easily, and tends not to eat enough, or they may be a child who never feels full. They may be a child who loves sweets or they may love salt. You need to respond to what your child brings. Later on they may be a child who uses food to comfort their emotions. You want to help them understand and manage their predispositions and tendencies in the unique times of plenty in which we live. An overemphasis on health may mean that you don't even notice or recognise these tendencies – that you are responding to your external agenda and not to the child in front of you.

The most important health matrix on food for children is 'enough'. The ubiquitous dieting culture means that we are steeped in a message that fewer calories is always a good thing, whereas kids need lots of calories, and often have limited palates (despite our best efforts), small appetites or short attention spans, and so we need to be careful that they eat enough. Parents can be driven to distraction or worry when their child isn't eating their lovingly prepared 'healthy' food, and whilst this is very frustrating, I would encourage any parent who experiences it to not allow a preoccupation with health to blind them to their child having enough food. I see many children and adolescents where a preoccupation with health in the family has contributed to them not eating enough. Many children aren't that bothered with food and will only eat stuff they really want.

Returning to my now grown son, as an adult, he eats pretty much everything. Indeed, his palate is very sophisticated, and he will eat all sorts of things I never offered at home. I don't think this was because of my 'perfect' weaning environment; nor do I think it is because I was firm in his childhood. The example I set at home may have been an influence – he's seen a balanced, morally neutral approach to all food – but probably, it's mostly because as he moved into teenage life he did want to go out with his mates, who ate a wider range of food, and he wanted to fit in.

THE GOOD-ENOUGH PARENT AND FEEDING YOUR CHILD

What does all this mean for you as you set out to wean your baby or feed your toddler? I guess it means that you can just be good enough, and not perfect: it means that you don't need to purée organic vegetables in a particular order. I would recommend not being too emotionally invested in the health angle of your child's food, but to consider it as one of many factors that are important about it – for example joy, variety and, most important of all, enough. You want to feed them based on the important nutritional information you have, including not getting so hung up on the quality of their calories that you forget to attend to the quantity being sufficient. But you want to be looking and listening to their intuition as well: what sort of eater are they? What do they like and not like? And can you help them expand that? Even with your best efforts, some children will be more 'fussy' than you want them to be: most do take in the major food groups (carbs, protein, fruit and veg), just without the range and flexibility you would want. There is a balance to be struck between offering them enough of the stuff they will eat, and also continuing to encourage the new stuff.

As they grow older, you want to raise them in an environment where all types of foods are available, and where the word 'healthy' is used judiciously. For me that meant always having biscuits, cakes and crisps in the house, so I could try to teach them restraint, but note my wording here: restraint, not restriction. Because in a context where all food is available, a smattering of restraint is required. Not eating something doesn't have to be because it's bad or banned or unhealthy. It can simply be about the concept of enough . . . 'I think you've probably had enough of that . . . how are you feeling? Are you still hungry?' In this way, you are encouraging them to tune in to their own internal drives and feelings, while also providing boundaries around nutrition. As they go into their tween and teenage years, they will provide boundaries around each other's eating in the guise of fairness: woe betide the sibling who eats more than their fair share of the biscuits.

The concept of balance can also be helpful. You want them to have a variety of food because that is psychologically and physically healthy. 'Can I have another biscuit, Mum?' can be answered with 'No. Two biscuits is enough.' Why is two enough? Well, you of course don't know exactly how much is intuitively satisfying to them, but you do roughly know about portion size, and that two of most snack things is probably enough. As they get older, you might want to explain that to them with 'I wouldn't want you to eat more than two apples at once. Eating too much of one thing is not a good thing.' You are not judging the food as good or bad – you are just encouraging balance. We know there is diminishing pleasure to food – our hedonic principle again: the third biscuit/apple is rarely as good as the first.

Finally, you can put some restrictions around their own intuition because you are not running a hotel, and do not need to provide exactly what they need or want on demand. So you could say, for example, 'No. You can't have more of that, because we had it yesterday/we're saving the rest for someone else/for tomorrow.' With my kids, who seemed to make a uteral pact not to like the same thing, they were allowed to leave some unfavoured foods at dinner, but otherwise they were expected to eat it all up. Don't go down the slippery slope of indulging everyone's whims with separate meals.

Some people are of the view that we should allow children to *only* depend on their intuition: they never put any restraint on what kids eat. But that wouldn't have worked for mine. Some kids will have a more naturally sweet tooth, have no sense of fullness and rarely feel fully satisfied. In our high-fat, high-sugar and processed food society, I don't think we can rely on intuition alone. There has to be a bit of parental common sense around children's nutrition at an early age, but just no morality, nor shaming about food. Those are the key tenets of nutrition and intuition.

In the academic literature, my concept of psychologically healthy, good-enough eating fits to that of 'responsive feeding in which a parent is attentive to a child's hunger and satiety cues, and monitors the quality of the child's diet' (see Table 1[xxxvii]). It continues, 'Thus, the challenge for caregivers is to provide structure and boundaries without decreasing children's eating autonomy to the extent that they no longer self-regulate their eating'.[xxxviii] I find the table below interesting, as it also outlines some of the common feeding pitfalls.

> **Table 1: Types of parent feeding from academic literature. Taken from Thompson, A.L. (2009).**
> 1) Laissez-faire, in which the parent does not limit infant diet quality or quantity and shows little interaction with the infant during feeding.
> 2) Pressuring/controlling, in which the parent is concerned with increasing the amount of food the infant consumes and uses food to soothe the infant.
> 3) Restrictive/controlling, in which the parent limits the infant to healthful foods and limits the quantity of food consumed.
> 4) Responsive, in which the parent is attentive to child hunger and satiety cues and monitors the quality of the child's diet.
> 5) Indulgent, in which the parent does not set limits on the quantity or quality of food consumed.

Your other framework tools – a reciprocal relationship and firm and kind – will help you provide a good-enough eating environment. Your reciprocity helps you tune in to their intuition and their other feelings. The goal of reciprocity is to help them listen to their own hunger and satiety, their preferences and tendencies and to guide them to balance these with broad ideas about nutrition. And you need some firmness and lots of kindness, because parents sometimes need to say (kindly), 'I expect you to try some fish' or, 'Don't eat all of that, please. There won't be any left for other people.' Or indeed, 'Are you feeling OK today?' But we do all that in a context of no restriction: of most food being available and provided.

Ideally, the good-enough parent demonstrates the nutrition–intuition balance in their own eating. As we have already discussed, children learn the most from observation of what we do, rather than what we say. It can be difficult for the parent who struggles with their own relationship with food and eating, but it is, of course, not a brilliant example if you are always yo-yo dieting or starting the latest trendy eating regime – if one week you are juicing and the next it's all about low-carb/cutting out all sugars/boring everyone with your Zoe data. Or oscillating between periods of rigid control, and then complete abandonment. I can remember one patient reflecting to me about her mum: 'She's always on a diet; she's been on a diet my whole life, but never seems to have lost any weight. I don't want to be like that.' Too often, I hear from patients that their parent (and sadly, it is usually the mum) doesn't eat family dinner. I feel compassion for these people, but raise the question of what sort of example this is. Do you want to teach your child that for their own life? Sometimes having kids can be the best motivation for sorting out your own shit: can you get some help here?

Two important concepts to demonstrate to our children are those of the tipping point and satiety. Food is generally a pleasure of diminishing returns; the first few mouthfuls are the best, and there is a tipping point when the pleasure starts to reduce: that is a good place to stop eating. Too often we are eating because the food is there in front of us, and we are chasing the enjoyment we got at the start. You want your children to see you stopping eating with delicious stuff still available: that you can do portion control. Satiety is about eating exactly what you fancy, in the right quantity and it being satisfying to you, so you don't need to eat more. Its opposite is eating something you don't really want 'because it's healthy' or that isn't quite enough, then ending up eating more later, as you were actually craving something different.

The good-enough parent tries to find the balance that is needed for health and satiety, ideally for themselves, and tries to demonstrate this for their child. They don't force any particular agenda down their child's throat – metaphorically and literally in this case. They know that we are all born with a natural preference for sweet and high fat, and that this needs some boundaries on it whilst kids are immature, but that trying to control it too much is counterproductive. Good-enough feeding provides both the traditionally 'healthy' and the not-so healthy food regularly, so that kids can observe, be encouraged and guided and, hopefully, find their own psychological balance in time. The good-enough parent also knows about the importance of food in a social context: the power of eating together, of food in culture, religion and celebration. They are mindful of our manifesto aims to feel joy in life, and that includes in food; not to be riddled with anxiety about it being healthy or fattening. They want emotionally competent kids, who have heard 'No, you can't have that' at times and have not had their every wish and whim indulged. But they also recognise their child may be a very different eater to them and are responsive to trying to understand that. Eventually, they'll want independent kids, so later, they will need to involve them in food preparation and cooking, and to take responsibility for that.

Ultimately, the good-enough parent knows that their child's eating is not in their control, nor is their future body shape. Those independent adults they are raising will have their own free will. Parents can demonstrate by example, eating joyfully with nutrition and intuition in mind, and providing a full food environment to try to teach their child the same.

FEEDING YOUR CHILD AND PERFECTIONISM

Food and eating are one of many areas where the perfect parent can become their own worst enemy. Whilst we are talking about food and eating in this chapter at the toddler age, this acts as an illustration of good-enough principles more generally, and the dangers when we shoot past good enough and try to be perfect. One of these important principles is being in a relationship with a child that is responsive to, but not dominated by them, whereby you help to guide their instincts and personality, rather than imposing a dogmatic, extreme standard upon them. The word that is often used for this is 'synchronicity'. Synchronicity loops right back to that attachment relationship – what we saw with the mother and baby in the Still Face Experiment (see p. 36). Perfectionists lose synchronicity because they are focused instead on an external standard and not the situation in front of them. And a lack of synchronicity between parent and child has been identified as one of the ways in which perfection can be potentially damaging to a child.

Parental expectations of perfection in food can become an intrinsic standard kids feel they have to meet, in the same way that they often feel they have to match behavioural or academic expectations. As always, though, perfectionism ignores the fact that your child is a different individual from you, and in the context of eating that will include their different patterns of hunger, preferences, fullness and satiety. It may lead to them becoming disconnected from their own intuition and nutritional needs in an effort to meet your standards. Through perfectionism children become disconnected from themselves.

Your job as a parent is not to mould your child into some version of best that is nothing like them. Nor to turn them into a mini you. Your job is to help them grow and develop into the best version of themselves, and that means understanding and responding to them: their own hunger and preferences, if we are talking about food and eating, but also in relation to different aspects of their individuality, which we will be thinking about later. Imposing a perfection ethos on your child is like trying to change a left-handed child to write with their right hand – you could probably do it if you really tried, but it is ultimately unhelpful.

PART 3: CHILDHOOD

3.1
The Busyness Business

It seems to me, when I meet my teenage patients, that the path of unhappiness that brought them to me was often established several years before, in their primary-school years. That might be a surprise to you, as it is typically seen as one of the least troubling stages of childhood, bookended by the trickier stages of toddler tantrums and teenage angst. But as you know, the teenagers I see often don't feel good enough, and when I trace back the roots of that feeling, more often than not, it seems to start in those middle-childhood years.

Children starting full-time education at the age of four in the UK begins a time of routine and consistency for most parents, where for thirty-nine weeks of the year, five days a week, your world is organised by the 9am and 3.30pm of the school day. Life becomes governed by the hours of the school day and the weeks of the school term and the terms of the school year. For some parents, this routine is a welcome relief or may mirror what they had set up for themselves in the baby and toddler years through nursery school or childcare. For others, it may feel like a loss of freedom, as the law suddenly has a say in what they do with their child. They are answerable to a headteacher about when they take their holidays, for example.

Either way, there is a sort of clarity to this part of parenting. Your role is consistent, regular. You deliver your child to school, you pick them up, you do their activities, you back up the school with reading and homework at home, you feed them and you get them to bed. And with that busy-ness, the days merge into weeks, the weeks into terms and the terms into years.

The business of busy-ness in childhood has become a big business. Activities that were once self-directed and kid-led have become clubs run by adults – from football to street dance. In the pursuit of excellence, anyone with a talent – such as sport or music – is singled out and trained up. Swimming, tennis and football clubs seem particularly keen to sign kids up into practice several times a week, leading to leagues and competitions. Whereas primary schools not so long ago would only send reading and times tables for homework, they now issue homework diaries and multiple tasks a week, and some of these involve a serious amount of adult support. Then, we have the explosion of private tutoring and tutoring companies – something that's become a multi-billion-pound business in one generation, it seems.[xxxix] We are trying to give our children the edge in an increasingly competitive world.

This is reflective of the glorification of hard work and busy-ness in society as a whole. 'Busy' has become a standard answer to the question 'how are you?' Politicians can't talk about families, without calling them 'hard-working families'. Do the families who work only moderately hard and have a good work–life balance not deserve consideration? Research into attitudes towards raising children since 1981 have asked the question: 'What values do we want in our children?'[xl] In 1990, in relation to the value of 'hard work', 29 per cent of people in the UK rated it as important; by 2022, this was 48 per cent.

Previously, in the absence of labour-saving devices, hard work was presumably necessary, but now it seems to have taken on a moral tone, and busyness is venerated or has come to signal 'important'. Similarly venerated is self-improvement, when in the past perhaps social attitudes towards class, and knowing your place, did not sit as easily with ideas about personal development. At school in the 1970s and 1980s, there was a relaxed attitude towards encouragement and achievement: I recently ran into an old art teacher who remembered my art as being really good and had kept photos of it. I just don't remember anyone telling me that at the time. There seems to have been much more of a belief in an immutable, innate ability rather than an encouragement to improve. Phrases like 'too big for their boots' reflected the importance of having a modest attitude to skills and talents.

Over the last generation, this seems to have changed, perhaps driven by the rise of individualism, as well as interest in early child development. By the time I had my first child in 2000, there was an emphasis on maximising children's ability. I can remember standing over my child's cot, fascinated in his interest in the black and white 'sensory' cloth books that were meant to stimulate his brain more than traditional cot bumpers or mobiles. Later, I invested in *Muzzy*, a BBC video series meant to give babies and toddlers exposure to a second language, and an advantage in learning one.[19] Carol Dweck's 2006 *New York Times* bestselling book on a growth mindset stressed to parents and teachers that, rather than seeing ability as fixed and innate, they needed to praise effort to enhance performance and give children a sense they could improve.[xli] Similarly, the idea of 10,000 hours of practice to become an expert, as popularised

---

19 It didn't work.

by Malcolm Gladwell in his *New York Times* bestselling book *Outliers*, was another part of this change in the narrative, stressing the importance of hard work over innate ability.[xlii, xliii] *Battle Hymn of the Tiger Mother*, published in 2011, became a handbook for ambitious parents looking for success for their children.

This is peak parenting-as-a-verb territory. If the only thing separating their child from success is an environment that nurtures it, parents set out to provide it, implicitly competing with each other for that success. The zeitgeist of this and the last generation, between schools, parents and society as a whole, has been a constant striving for the child to achieve the best. Nobody could argue against this as a goal, right? You want the best for your child.

Well, I do wonder if the pendulum has now swung too far. There seems to be a myth that hard work conquers all. We have indoctrinated kids in a belief that it is just their own personal effort that will determine their outcome. Stories like that of *King Richard*, telling how the dad of the Williams sisters plotted their careers, contribute to the belief that parents can plan success, if they are just committed enough. In parents' minds, sometimes all that is standing in the way of their child's success is hard work and commitment. We see them all as potential Olympians or Juilliard artists. We overlook the role of raw talent and luck.

There's a Gary Lineker YouTube video called 'Shut up and let them play' that is worth watching, on parents' unrealistic expectations of their children's football skills. Gary recounts how, when on the touchline, watching his own sons playing football, he saw another parent yell in their child's face as he came off the pitch: 'If you play like that, you are never going to make the grade'. Gary said he thought, 'Mate, I've watched him play. He ain't gonna make the grade anyway, so just chill. Let him enjoy his football.' He goes on to say, 'The truth is they'll reach the level that they reach anyway. [With that pressure] they are much less likely if they had an inkling of a possibility of making it, they are decreasing those chances.'[xliv]

When most successful people talk about their success, they always seemingly want to justify it by stressing how hard they worked. In fact, 99 per cent of boys signed to a premier-league academy at nine years old will not have a professional footballing career, and I'm sure that most of them work their socks off. I'm sure they want it as much, and give their all. They likely just aren't as good at the time, or don't get lucky. But the hard-work-and-effort-conquer-all myth may contribute to the shame and mental-health difficulties that many of them suffer when dropped.[xlv]

The emphasis on effort over ability, the belief that hard work conquers all, contributes to a childhood based on outcome. Before this information age, our ancestors may have expected their children to work the fields or in factories towards a product or output. But now, the child's behaviour and achievements *are* the product or output. Their swimming, piano, drama, maths, English, attendance, cycling proficiency, classroom tidiness, healthy lunchboxes, behaviour, weight and all are marked by certificates, badges, charts, grades and tests. We saw the beginnings of this in toddler years with the numerous tasks on a star chart, and we risk that in these middle-childhood years it gets more intense, our children's output being measured and monitored as carefully as product control on the assembly line, by the state, the education system and ourselves, as parents. There is this constant race towards better. We say, 'That's brilliant ... and next time, stretch a bit further/practise a bit longer/do this extra training'. Rarely is it said, 'He is doing enough. He's great, there is nothing extra he needs to do.'[20] A childhood literally and metaphorically marked off through comparative and competitive activities. The great psychotherapist and author Julia Samuel said it best to me once: it is a commodification of childhood.

I think we need to find that messy middle again. Hard work and support are important to success, but so are talent, luck and, most of all, timing. Ten thousand hours' practice is a necessary condition for expertise, but it is not the only one. Indeed, Gladwell's analysis also focuses on how success is intrinsically linked to unique opportunities of ability meeting historical timing: being there at the right time with the right unique skills. That Bill Gates not only did 10,000 hours of practice but was in the right place at the right time. Instead, we seem to have moved to a position of extreme parenting: an arms race of time invested in children's potential, parents competing for their offspring's apparent genius.

TIPPING POINTS FOR BUSY-NESS?
In thinking about how to be a parent during these childhood years, I want us to be reminded of one of our aims: we want them to feel good enough during their teenage and adult years. Perhaps you believed that to build children's confidence, you need to give them lots of opportunities to achieve and have those achievements marked and celebrated. To, in fact, give them as many activities as you can possibly afford and manage. Well, I don't think so.

---

20 As I write this, I realise that I've written 'stretch/ed' twice in one paragraph and so I look to the thesaurus for some synonyms. Do you know what the synonyms are for 'stretch/ed'? Stressed, struggling, fraught, overextended. What are we doing to our young people?

Many of the kids I see in clinic have extensive extra-curricular, adult-led timetables, full of activities that they reportedly love, but which, collectively, leave them strung out and exhausted. Parents, perhaps secretly hopeful of their child's inherent genius, justify the extra-curricular routine and the expense because their child loves dance, drama, ju-jitsu , whatever.

But it seems that parents have forgotten to say enough is enough. It's not just the good we need to focus on in our good-enough parenting – it's the enough. More of a good thing isn't always better; more is sometimes worse. There is a tipping point. It is worse, for example, when it starts to overstimulate kids, when there is no downtime and free play or when it stresses or exhausts parents. When it gets in the way of relationships. Or when I have parents desperate to bring their distressed child to see me, but they can't find any time between the swimming, tutoring, orchestra and running club. Their child is unhappy, possibly even self-harming, but it seems impossible for them to step off the achievement-travelator for long enough to see a mental-health professional.

But there is a second tipping point. When children are engaged in adult-supervised activity, and we (parents, coaches, teachers) give our feedback, we risk making kids too invested in our opinion. This second tipping point is created within the child, where an opportunity a parent is giving them starts to feel like an expectation on them that they have to fulfil. Over time, it can stop being something they are doing for themselves, because they love it, and instead, something that is tied to others' perceived opinions. Children can get hooked on praise and admiration, and they don't want to let anyone down. We risk linking their activity to the external validation (praise, stars, certificates; people pleasing), rather than their internal feelings (joy, fun and pride in taking part). A sense of self-esteem based on other people's opinions, on doing well, winning, getting those ticks and stars, is a bucket with a hole in it. The more achievement you put in at the top, the more it pours out the bottom, and you seemingly need more success to keep any inside.

I often use Taylor Swift's words with my patients, as she seems to capture this experience of young people really well: that of the archetypal 'good girl' or 'people pleaser'. In her documentary *Miss Americana* she speaks about how she was trained through childhood and adolescence to look for the approval of others – 'those pats on the head were all I lived for'. She charts the process of giving this up and becoming her own person, rather than the one everyone else wanted her to be.

I want to digress a moment here and be clear about what I'm *not* saying. I'm not saying we shouldn't give kids opportunities – kids at this age are like sponges, absorbing new information, picking up new skills, developing more talents. Nor am I saying that we shouldn't place any expectations on our kids. It is reasonable to have expectations of their behaviour, manners and values. What I am saying here – and throughout the book – is that we just need to be careful: first, with the sheer number of expectations and what is developmentally appropriate, *and* with outcome-based expectations, where their involvement becomes *our* pride, rather than *their* joy.

Of course, your kids should do some activities; Michelle Obama was, as usual, wise on this, saying that her daughters had one activity for themselves and one that was decided by their parents. Mostly, the kinds of opportunities we need to give them are ones they would seek out if they were left with limited adult intervention . . . the kind they do for the pure joy of doing them. If you didn't take them to Harriers club, would they be making up running races with their friends and siblings? Are you forcing them into music or are they drawn towards it?

Are they a kid who seeks out maths problems for fun? This also seems to have been missed in Gladwell's stories of success: the successful, yes, had a nurturing environment. They had a nurturing environment *for their own particular obsession or interest*: it was supported by adults, but not enforced by them. The challenge is to spark their passion not to impose your own.

This busy-ness starts in primary-school years but does not show its toxic tentacles till later. Whilst some kids struggle with attention or behaviour at this age, most pootle along happily enough with the adult agenda. They are, on average, more compliant than they are in the toddler or teenage stages: they may argue about piano practice or Kumon maths, but mostly, they do not down tools, as they will both earlier and later. But is the damage being done in how we are training them to always be trying to be better or want more: are we setting up the belief in them, in effect, that they have to achieve to be worthy of love? Although children at this age don't protest, when I see them in tween years, there is a shift. They don't articulate it clearly, but it seems that tipping point has passed and the opportunities *for* them have morphed into expectations *of* them in their minds. The activity they once loved has started to be a thing on a to-do list of self-improvement.

When I see teenage patients, they are so often strung out with other people's opinions on every aspect of their existence. Even when they are the most successful, with a string of A*s, Grade 8 music or places at 'top' universities, no achievement is ever enough; there is always more that they could do. Another step they need to take along the adult-approved path, which has now often become internalised in their own psyche.

THE BUSYNESS AND MANIFESTO AIMS

As they enter their middle-childhood years, with all this busy-ness, we risk starting them on a path that is inconsistent with manifesto aims. As parents, we can end up communicating a constantly striving, always-tweaking, could-be-better mentality to our kids, which is replicated in education and on the internet. In the next chapter, we will look at how the school system has become overly focused on grades and qualifications and is testing kids into relentless, hamster-wheel work schedules or a sense of failure. And yes, it is also happening via everyone's favourite scapegoat – the internet and the phone: what starts as a means of communication and fun games can become a black hole of comparison. Ironically, kids use their screens to escape the demands on them in the real world, but there they find a whole heap of different, possibly more alluring options-for-improvement.

A path of busyness for a child can lead to a cage of standards and expectations for an adolescent. Growing up with a constant narrative of self-improvement from the surrounding adults can lead a child into either perfectionism themselves or disenfranchise them into rebellion. We will be talking about the rebellious adolescent more in the next chapters, but the type of perfectionism I mean here is a particularly toxic type called socially prescribed perfectionism. This is not about having your own intrinsically high standards, but rather a sense of being judged and graded all the time, of constantly worrying about the opinion of others. This leaves people feeling disconnected not only from their own motivation and enthusiasm, but sometimes from any sense of their own wishes, feelings and opinions at all. Socially prescribed perfectionism keeps young people trapped in social convention, in other people's standards of best: it is strongly associated with feeling sad, lonely and anxious, and the associated mental-health conditions. Over the last few decades, socially prescribed perfectionism has increased amongst college students, and this has been linked to the perfectionism in parenting and schools.[xlvi]

So this section of the book looks upstream from adolescence – the primary-school years. How does the good-enough parent give opportunities to their child without riddling their adolescent with self-defeating expectations in the future? How do they allow their child to grow and develop themselves, and not mould them into their version of best? In the next three chapters of the book, we will look at the education system, and how you support your children to meet their potential comfortably. We will also look at your child's relationships, and how you maintain your own relationship with them, whilst also supporting them in spreading their wings into new friendships. And we will look at the internet, and how to set the boundaries your child needs to use it safely.

The relationship piece is particularly important. You see, I don't just think the busy-ness business is dangerous because it lodges relentless standards in a child's head. I also think it is damaging in another way. In creating a busy childhood, with multiple activities and undue importance placed on academic outcome, we risk raising kids in a high-pressure, rushed environment. Fitting in all this busy-ness becomes a scheduling nightmare, with us rushing in and barking at our kids to get ready for the next thing, and have they done their homework, spellings, times-table practice? Have they had their healthy snack? Now hurry-hurry-hurry, on to the next thing. It risks making us so stretched and busy that we never stop and smell the roses. Or, more specifically, sit and play Lego. Or sit at all, really, as there is always somewhere to go and something to do. We risk, as parents, investing so much in our children that we *expect* an outcome from them, as we do when we buy something in a shop or restaurant, and feeling frustrated when they are not up to standard, or getting with the programme. In doing this, we risk damaging our relationship with them.

We are going to think about how a good-enough parent does not impose too much of their dreams on their child and protects them from the overvaluing of busy-ness by others when they can, supporting them to take them with a pinch of salt when they can't. And whilst hard work is an important value, I want you to remember there are other values available: joy, happiness, connection, fun, adventure, kindness, creativity, flexibility, acceptance, relaxation . . . We are going to think about how you don't sacrifice all the other values on the altar of hard work and busyness.

Because here's the nub. The way we create a sense of 'good enough' in kids is not by giving them achievements, accomplishments and outcomes. No, we create this through our relationship with them, giving a sense of warmth and attachment during their childhood. And if all that busy-ness doesn't leave enough time, money or energy to give them warmth, then it is counterproductive.

We need to try to value them just the way they are; who they are, not who we want them to be. And do you know what happens when we value people the way they are? They often use this as a secure base to jump off to the next step.

3.2
School and Education

The main arena the busyness business gets played out in is educating children. There are many players here: the government, the media, education authorities, chains and academy trusts, universities, colleges and employers, schools, headteachers, teachers, tutors and parents. At the centre of all this busyness is a child. A child who needs to learn some stuff.

In my opinion, the system of education in the UK and in numerous countries around the world, has two major flaws. Firstly, it is contributing to the mental-health problems of many. Secondly, it is not helping a lot of young people into appropriate work. I believe that both these flaws are because the education systems have become less about education and more about qualifications. I do not see this as the fault of the many good and dedicated school staff or parents who want to help children fulfil their potential. I see a lot of the players as unwitting cogs in a wheel. Schools are pressurised and lured to become qualification factories – to get kids through exams and into the next factory – and feted as the 'best' school when they do so, whatever the costs for children.

How parents are in relation to their child's education can, again, be seen through the good-enough continuum: some parents do not support their child's learning enough; some have a balanced approach and some are too tied in to their child's academic success. I am conscious that, since I started out as a clinical psychologist and a parent, I've moved backwards and forwards on this continuum. At the start, I probably was pretty much in the middle: I thought my children would end up at a good-enough school, preferably close to our home, and do fine, as I had.

However, as I spoke and listened to other parents, and looked into results tables for local schools, I started to realise that there had been a seismic change in the way we educate kids since I was at school – a change that is driven by results, emphasises standardisation and involves frequent evaluation. I also saw that many parents were targeting their churchgoing, house buying and work lives according to perceptions of what were the best schools. Parents were all getting more involved, focused on maximising potential and giving children as many opportunities as possible – what I now call outcome-based parenting. There was almost a frenzy about it, a fear-based narrative that if you didn't do this, your child would miss out or have to settle for second best in the mass competition of life. I fell into that black hole for a while. I thought of schools and education just in terms of academic achievement; I actively sought out 'best' schools. And I think back with shame about the time I queried a teacher on why my six-year-old wasn't making the expected progress, as if he were a piece of meat going into a sausage machine, due to come out perfectly uniform. I think, now, parental anxiety about doing the best for my child made me swing way past good enough, and want better and more. It made me forget what I knew about child development and blind to the costs of a striving mindset.

Yes, I fell into the perfectionist, outcome-based hole for a few years in raising my children vis-à-vis education, and it might have continued had I not had the privilege of listening to older children and adolescents every day in my work and hearing about the immense cost to them of their education. Oh, of course, they didn't say it like that. My anxious, sad, eating-disordered and self-harming patients instead said things like, 'We got our revision booklets for our SATs', 'Our head of year gave us a talk that we needed to work harder this year than ever before' and, 'They won't let me drop my fourth A level'. Then they told me of their relentless work schedules and fear of failure, which often meant a B or C, and their desire to 'do well', which often meant being at the very top. After their exams, I would see them again, thinking that some of them might be content now with having achieved their success, but no, they were just kind of, well, to use their word, 'meh'. There was a deep-seated unease about what was it all for. Or an embedded sense of failure that, given they had dropped one grade on one subject, they were no longer going to the course or university they had been encouraged to dream of. There seemed few winners in this system.

I began to get curious about what was going on here. I became a school governor, and I started writing for an educational journal about mental health and judging schools for wellbeing initiatives on a national level. I learnt a lot. In this way, I swung back to the middle to find my good-enough balance, based on a realistic appraisal of where we are now, and I hope I can help you find yours, too.

THE POLITICAL BECOMES PERSONAL: CHANGES IN EDUCATION
Forgive me if I digress for a moment and talk about the changes that have happened in the education system over the last forty years. They may feel irrelevant to you, but I believe they are as important in understanding the crisis in young people's mental health as the digital revolution that we will be talking about

later. They have happened in plain sight, but we are somehow blind to them. They are something I could bang on about for half a book, and indeed, you must thank my editors that I am not.

In education around the world there has been a move to standardise teaching, and increase the focus on core subjects, assessment of children and the inspection of schools. Schools have entered a free-market economics framework, encouraging competition between them and giving an illusion of parental choice. These changes have been referred to as the Global Education Reform Movement, or GERM. The term was coined by Paul Sahlberg to capture a phenomenon of how the education systems, starting in the UK and US, reformed in a particular style, and how that style spread, as germs do, around the world[xlvii].

There are many examples of how this has happened but let me give you one from England and Wales. In 1988, a series of educational reforms created a National Curriculum of stuff that schools should teach. I'm pretty sure that these reforms were brought in with good intention – that the politicians and policy makers were aiming to improve standards and ensure every child got a good education. Indeed, I think we needed these reforms; for example, I always remember an administrator at a school telling me about how, before the National Curriculum, the Year 2 teacher used to strum his guitar most of the day, with singing and music forming most of his self-determined curriculum for that year. A standardised curriculum was needed to prevent situations like this and ensure all children were getting a consistent education.

Quite reasonably, to check that the schools followed this law and taught what had been mandated by government, some standardised assessment tests were introduced: the

Year 6 SATs. However, over the next few years, comparative SAT results for each school began to be published in national newspapers. And in this way, over time, they became not a measure of how well the school was teaching the National Curriculum, but rather a test of how good the school was. And that changed everything. The tests have become high stakes for the school, the head, the teachers, and this pressure inevitably trickles down the system to the parents and the children. Revision booklets are sent out; Easter work is organised; kids compare themselves to their peers; practice papers are sold in local corner shops. The whole school needs to be quiet when the Year 6 children are sitting their SATs. Kids are indoctrinated into the belief that this *matters* in some way. That this will somehow impact their futures in some indeterminable way: that they are or aren't clever; or will or won't do well, or be successful.

And in this example, we start to see some of the risks of the GERM: how good intentions to improve misfire into a narrowing of the curriculum, an individualised pressure, a competitive-comparative attitude which can be harmful to kids. It also hints at the spiralling that can happen: an arms race, where each year schools try to 'improve standards', with the admirable purpose to 'help every child reach their potential' or 'maximise their opportunities'. But there doesn't seem to be a limit on that; it's like, globally, we are saying to children, 'Well done, you ran a four-minute mile. Now let's go for the three-minute mile.' We don't seem to acknowledge that there are limits to our children's learning abilities. The GERM was needed but has spread way past good enough to become an infection of perfection. Now some might say that the kids need to toughen up; that's what the real world is like. But in fact, this doesn't seem to prepare kids for adult life; it contributes instead to the situation we have now, where many are zoned out or burnt out by education.

It seems that education is much more at the whim of the beliefs of the politicians of the day. Successive governments reform the system in the image of their own personal success. I became aware of this when I was both working in the NHS in a hospital and as a governor at a school 1 mile away. I noticed a contrast in the two settings in that government certainly fiddled with the bureaucracy and organisation in the medical setting, but they did not determine how we treated our patients – that would depend on scientific research. But it seems politicians think they know best about how to educate kids, be that quotas for tertiary education, selection at eleven years old or rote learning of historical facts.[21] Their arrogance allows actual evidence on the success of less comparative, competitive education systems (such as Finland) to be ignored.

So as a parent thinking about schools and learning, I implore you to think about how much you embrace the system or whether you take it with a pinch of salt. Or a bucketload.[22]

BEING A GOOD-ENOUGH PARENT IN EDUCATION

How does the good-enough parent keep their head in all this? Where is the messy middle in starting your educational journey with your children? Let's return to the continuum.

We know that children who are not supported at all in education do less well. That if their parents don't value education, if they have no role models of success in their environment and if their parents are not ambitious for their future, this is

---

21 For these examples, Margaret Thatcher, Tony Blair, Theresa May and Michael Gove spring to mind.
22 Some of the people writing and talking about education who have influenced me are Alfie Kohn, Ken Robinson, Paul Sahlberg.

not a good thing in terms of educational outcome. What is less discussed is that some kids don't do as well at school because their intrinsic level of intelligence is lower, or they are not so good at the academic curriculum or aren't interested. A qualification-based education system risks focusing too little on these kids. Yet school should be a good experience for everyone – one that embeds them into a community and society as a whole. Shouldn't future fruit pickers and shelf stackers be as much valued in the education system as nuclear scientists and brain surgeons? We need all of them invested in society for it to work.

But at the other end of our good-enough continuum, extreme parenting can take the support we should be offering to our children in school to the nth degree. Parents seemingly get sucked into a vortex that values educational performance, academic success and excellence above all, and life revolves around school and schoolwork. I've never seen any parent who thinks they are doing this, and, if asked directly, they will always say that they just want their child to be happy and healthy. But seemingly, they must believe that the route to that happiness is through academic achievement, because their actions (their time, money and energy) strongly suggest they value education the most.

So whilst it is undoubtedly a good thing to have interested, involved parents, what I see echoes what we have also seen with food and activities: that there is a point where this parental support and ambition tip into unhelpful. I have seen too many parents who seemingly forget to balance any other aspect of parenting alongside the focus on education. They forget that parent is a noun about a relationship, as they actively try to parent their child into success. It infiltrates every part of life: the conversations they have with their children, organising, structuring and supervising homework, reading, tutoring, discussions about the future. Getting ahead, doing more, getting better.

Of course, parents are reflective of society. When I was raising my children in the early part of this century, I kept hearing about how our kids would be competing against those from India and China in a global economy. We have constant headlines about school performance, exam results, standards in schools and competition for university places. Perfectionism is an anxious state at the best of times; a perfectionistic parent can worry about a hundred things in the comfort of their own home with their babe safe in their arms. But put their child in global competition with a scarcity mindset of only so many places at the top table, and the perfectionist parent will implode with anxiety; and when people feel anxious, they often try to take control of things. They put more effort into trying to micro-manage their child's outcome, and so pressure in the whole system amplifies.

The anxious, perfectionistic parent, or the good-enough parent who is having an off day, tries to control and manage. They try to get ahead of the curve, and on the fast-track trajectory that they believe will take their child to success and happiness. The perfectionistic mindset finds the vulnerable reality that we do not control our children's outcomes unbearable. They try to ensure, through the sheer force of their determination, the power of their organisational skills and the investment in the best resources, that they get their kid 'the best' in life.

In my work, I've seen adolescents who have seemed broken by the academic demands put on them, kids who have stopped going to school – they are often bright, bold, defiant, but they are seemingly paralysed by the dissonance between the expectations on them and their capacity to fulfil them. Countless girls who regularly self-harm, but are so indoctrinated into a system of upward trajectory and self-improvement that they would sincerely believe they were 'failing' if they got a B. That pressure feels so awful in their heads and hearts that the only way they can think of to assuage it is to take a razor to their arms. I've seen adolescents incapacitated by anxiety, not sleeping, not eating and, again and again, when I unpick the mentally ill thoughts underlying their distress it is this same mantra: they don't feel good enough. If I had a pound for every time a mentally unwell teenager had said to me, 'My teacher will be disappointed in me' to justify a punishing work schedule . . . They are terrified to step off the hamster wheel for one minute. Of course, schoolwork isn't the only factor (we will get to the bogeyman of screen use soon), but it is clear to me that it is a major contributory factor to the pressure.

I would see adolescents suffering like this, all day, and then go to pick my kids up from their primary school 1 mile away from the hospital where I worked. In the playground, parents would come to talk to me, as a psychologist and school governor, about their concerns about their children or the school. One was worried about their kid's academic progress: he wasn't reading yet, and they wanted to get him into a good school. One bemoaned the lack of calligraphy and Shakespeare. I did try to take their concerns seriously, but after a day spent mentally patching up the adolescent victims of this type of mindset, I, like Gary Lineker, also wanted to say, 'Stop, please stop. Please do not put pressure on them in primary school. Let them play. Let them pootle around. Let them explore learning, go at their own pace, be curious and not judged. Let them gain confidence and feel good enough. Let's not embed them in a system of doing better and getting more at this early age.' I wanted to shout it from the rooftops.

ACADEMIC STRIVING AND THE MANIFESTO

Again, a pause to think about what I am *not* saying: I am not saying academic success or qualifications aren't important; nor that they don't depend in part on hard work, as well as a heap of other factors, including innate ability and luck. And, of course, I believe parents should be interested and support kids in their learning; but they should be mindful that they are in a global system of pressure already, and think about whether they amplify or mitigate that pressure. My advice is to focus on your children's actual academic output judiciously and sparingly. Let's have a think about this through the lens of our manifesto aims.

We'll start with the manifesto aim of being independent and capable. Nowadays, many children are working to fulfil their potential like a premier-league footballer does: with the full back-up of support staff – in this case, their parents, tutors, holiday courses, online resources. Parents have a full workload of scheduling, planning, getting their snack, and helping with homework. Some children then end up being a whizz at quadratic equations but having never made a cup of tea. The risk here is that a child is either deprived of the sense of pride and purpose that comes from completing a task independently or from learning from their own mistakes. Too much parental involvement risks giving them inflated expectations of themselves in the future, that can lead to the paralysis of perfection, where it becomes a catastrophe when they don't get an A. When parents (and their paid accomplices, tutors) are very involved in a child's learning, it ends up breeding dependence, rather than independence. I have also seen many young people who continue to need that external help to get through university, or in their jobs. Emerging adults are left with imposter syndrome, as their 'success' is built on the extensive support of others.

Over-investing in your child's academic performance also impacts on the manifesto aim to have a good relationship with them. Because if you parent like this, you also give up part of your relationship as a parent to be that teacher. When you instinctively greet them after school with 'How did you do in your spelling test?' or some other academic enquiry, you are not leading with social, emotional and practical parent stuff, but with teacher stuff. You risk undermining the most important thing you can give your child: unconditional love. Now, of course I know you do love your child unconditionally, but do *they* know it? Because when you shine that metaphorical attention lamp on your head on to their academic performance – or its absence – you risk giving them a belief that their worth and value in life depend on this. Relationship-based parenting leads with the relationship, not their performance or output. It knows that fun, relaxation, downtime, chatting-over-a-biscuit-time are as important as reading together, practising spellings and doing times tables.

Focusing on academic performance is also, by its very nature, future-focused – whether on the next test, doing the homework, making the grade – and the GERM agenda has exacerbated this with its overreliance on rigorous, repetitive testing. As parents, if we buy into this too much, we over-sacrifice the present for the future, and risk creating that striving, anxious state that Jonny Wilkinson described: looking for future happiness through suffering. This is the opposite of our manifesto aim of having low-anxiety kids. Parents often think they are getting kids into good habits by expecting excellence on their homework, tests and exams, even in the early years, but I find that this often creates anxiety in the diligent and a zoning out in the less diligent. We need to develop a low-anxiety state in ourselves: a belief that our kid will get there in the end and they don't need to be getting top marks when they are in primary school.

Our manifesto aim of happiness is associated with being present in the here and now; being able to see the pleasure of the moment. Children naturally think about the present. It is one of the most charming and frustrating things about them – that they stop in the street to show you a snail or a pretty leaf, when you are rushing to get to school on time. As parents and in education, we seem to be relentlessly trying to train them out of this, to be, instead, future-focused; and then, in adolescence, when they are stressed and unhappy, we try to teach them mindful skills to be in the moment! This is crazy. We need instead to embed their capacity to be in the moment in these early years; to allow space for it, time to give them good memories, which provides a pattern for their future happiness and an expectation of wanting this in life. We do not control what will happen to them in life, but a capacity for joy prepares them better for all the difficulties they will inevitably face and provides counterbalance and recovery if they choose a life of hard work in the future.

And what about good enough? Does the academic agenda give them a sense of being good enough? A future-focused, outcome-based childhood never allows for them being fine where they are. It is always focusing on the next thing. When parents get very involved in their child's work and stretch them to do the very best they can, they are often creating an expectation that their child works beyond their actual, comfortable capacity. We try to create the attitude of an Olympic champion adult in a child; in a child doing a craft homework. There has been a bastardisation of the phrase 'do your best', which used to mean 'try hard for a bit', but now seems to have morphed to mean 'work to your maximum capacity, till exhaustion'. The 10,000-hours-practice hypothesis was, in the original research, about becoming expert in a particular skill, not about being excellent at everything. Expecting excellence at all times in all things leads to burnout or zone-out. Where is the concept of good-enough work?

And finally, emotional competence. Resilience is a very popular word in the child-development space, and the idea that we create resilience by giving children hard experiences. Perhaps the academic focus and the hard work are the route to this? No, that seems to keep many children in a state of constant tension, with no recoil, until by adolescence any elastic potential is gone. I don't think the route to emotional competence is the micro-managed, parent-supervised path to academic success. Rather, it's children having a range of different experiences which they either manage themselves or choose to share with you. Free play in the park with their friends, where someone falls over and two people fall out. Managing their homework themselves – forgetting it and getting into minor trouble with their teacher and hiding that from you. Low-stakes problems that they resolve themselves are a more likely path to emotional competence.

THE MENTAL-HEALTH COSTS OF ACADEMIC PRESSURE
Children who are under a lot of academic pressure show up in mental-health or other support services in my experience in two main ways.

They can show up a lot in adolescence, having quietly absorbed and complied with the busyness agenda for years, and with anxiety, eating disorders or self-harm. This group is largely girls. We will return to them in Chapter 4.1, 'The Perfect Storm', but upstream of this, in childhood, parents should be aware of how pressure in these middle-childhood years can play out later. In brief, school and academic pressure is consistently seen in the data as one of the main factors that is breaking our adolescents. We know children and adolescents are getting more unhappy. In the financial year 2021–2, 1.2 million children were referred to the NHS Child and Adolescent Mental Health Services in England – that runs at about 18 per cent of all possible six- to seventeen-year-olds.[23] [xlviii, xlix] There is consistent data linking this unhappiness to school and schoolwork in adolescence. The Children's Society Good Childhood annual survey has shown that children report they are specifically unhappy with schoolwork, and their happiness on this issue has decreased over the last ten years.[l] In the UK, our fifteen-year-olds show up as feeling amongst the most pressurised with schoolwork in World Health Organization data.[li]

But here in the childhood section of the book, we are going to focus on the other way they show up, and that is at around six or seven years old, because they are not making the educational grade in some way. This group is largely boys. This is when school settings get serious about kids sitting still, and so, perhaps encouraged by outcome-focused schools, parents are looking for educational or behavioural assessments to explain how and why their child is not keeping up with their peers with, for example, a query diagnosis of ADHD or dyslexia.

When children are not making the grade, even though parents have moved to a new area to get them into that high-achieving school, or are paying for a top school, there is a tendency to look

---

[23] In the younger ages, boys outnumber girls and the pattern reverses in older adolescents. Mental-health rates amongst teenage girls run at 25 per cent. Struggling boys show up in youth justice figures more frequently than girls.

for a label to help explain that. Society's glorification of academic achievement contributes to no parent liking to think that their child is less intelligent than average. I feel uncomfortable even writing this – like I am dissing those kids – but of course, if there is an average, some children have to be below it. And yet, whilst plenty of parents come to me saying that their child is the messiest, the most disobedient, even the most unwell, none has ever said to me 'My child isn't intelligent'. They'll say, 'They are really smart, but they have dyslexia/dyscalculia/dyspraxia/executive-functioning problems/ADHD/sensory-processing difficulties' (delete as applicable).

Reading, maths, writing, spelling, attention, motivation, etc. are all skills that may or may not come easily and early for your children. They may fall behind their peers on any of these in primary years, because schools are set up for an average ability and for steady progress. In fact, it is completely normal for children to progress at different speeds and to have different abilities; in time, children either catch up, and/or they will also likely find their own path, which probably won't be the thing that they found difficult. Yet, the education system is structured around average progress, and parents can get a message that their child is not achieving and look for an explanation for this, and so take their child for an educational or behavioural assessment.

Early on in my career, I did a huge number of these, both in the community and as part of a comprehensive assessment in a children's psychiatric unit. In them, we are not searching for an actual definitive thing in the way that a doctor might look at an X-ray for a broken bone. We are looking for a mismatch between a child's general intelligence level (their IQ) or their age and their performance on a particular test or range of tests. This is more akin to a doctor looking at an X-ray to compare a child's bone size or growth to what is normal for children of their age. When we see such a mismatch, we can give a label to it – dyslexia or ADHD, for example. When I worked in a psychiatric hospital, it was amazing how many children got to the point of psychiatric admission without realising that they had this sort of learning difficulty that was impacting on their mood and behaviour, setting them on the trajectory that led them to them being admitted. Often, these children were economically or socially deprived and did not have the sort of parents who knew how to advocate for them. An adequate assessment and support package in the community could have perhaps prevented their admission.

So I think educational assessments can be helpful, if not essential, for fully understanding difficulties, but, as with many of the issues in this book, the problems arise at both ends of the good-enough continuum: with under-diagnosis, as we see here, and with over-diagnosis.

Over-diagnosis is an area where we need to be careful that parenting doesn't go to extremes. Because in this qualification-obsessed society, there is a hell of a lot of over-testing and over-labelling of children whose parents who can afford it. Parents looking for an explanation or to support their child can end up taking them for many different assessments. When they do that, the chances of finding something 'wrong' are increased because these diagnoses are hazy and overlapping and because there is immense variation in ability in all of us. I think if you assessed any child for long enough, you could find something in them that they were bad at. This is why a higher number of pupils receive extra time and rest breaks in exams in private schools, as opposed to the state schools, despite many of them being academically selective.[lii] The system can certainly be exploited by those who can pay. But such over-testing and over-labelling can also be an unhelpful way to parent: a different form of our extreme parenting. So the good-enough parent should be wary of too much assessment.

A key point with these diagnoses is that we have no way of knowing whether they reflect a significant long-term difficulty or a delay in picking up some skills. This may be a stable thing, i.e. something a child is bad at when they are ten years old and will continue to be bad at all their life. Or it may be something that they are just a bit slow in picking up but will get in adult life. As an analogy, I found learning to drive inordinately difficult. I started driving in a little Jeep on my grandparents' farm and, for some reason (undiagnosed 'dyspraxia', probably), I steered into rather than away from animals, fences, hedges. It was terrifying. When it was my brother's turn, he did it naturally. Then, when I was allowed on the roads, I still struggled and needed endless driving lessons. But eventually, I got it. I reached the standard required for the test and have driven around safely enough ever since. Almost certainly, if we tested my intrinsic skill level, it would not be good enough for me to be a Formula 1 driver, but it is good enough for the life I lead. Similarly, these diagnoses sometimes reflect a lifelong and intrinsic difficulty and sometimes a developmental delay, which your child will catch up on in time and reach a good-enough level for adult life.

One of the troubles with a diagnosis is it can be used as a catch-all; there is a tendency these days for any strength or difficulty to be subsumed into these terms. Using dyslexia as an example, it is, at its core, a mismatch between reading ability and chronological age/general IQ. But what I see, in clinic and online, is that it is used as an umbrella term seemingly to capture every aspect of a young person's functioning: creativity, memory strengths or weaknesses, attention.[liii] A diagnosis can be a springboard to aid understanding, access help or to guide future growth, but, in a world where young people have too much pressure and expectation on them, it can be used as a safety blanket or as a way to explain every quirk in their behaviour or performance – an excuse-all, get-out-of-jail-free card: 'I can't do that because of my dyslexia/sensory processing/dyscalculia'. Typical of this is an online post I saw the other day, in which a young person described an incredibly busy, stressful day (a day anyone would have found exhausting) and how she forgot that 'because of her ADHD', she needed to rest. With the glorification of achievement and worshipping at the altar of qualifications, has rest become only justifiable through a neurodiversity?

So the good-enough parent has to be careful of over-assessment and over-labelling, and giving kids a narrative whereby they believe they have something innate and permanently wrong with them. Rather, we want an attitude of compassionate understanding that we all have strengths and weaknesses, and the latter are opportunities for growth. Vis-à-vis the manifesto aim of making a child feel they are good enough, understanding their difficulties can be helpful, but there is a point where it becomes self-defeating; where we are giving children a problem-saturated childhood: where everything revolves around their difficulties.

The system (you, as parents, and your child's school) should be able to absorb a range of speeds and abilities, offering the necessary patience and support for children to learn skills at their own pace. Kids may need extra teaching time to overcome any academic (reading, writing or maths) struggles, but if your child is below average, avoid *overly* focusing on what they are not very good at. I see so many parents who worry that their child will have low self-esteem if they don't catch up to the majority, and they do a deep dive into intensive 'treatments' that actually have little evidence base. Currently, there is a tendency to try to over-teach, seeing every interaction as a potential learning opportunity, which will damage your relationship and likely put your child off. Children see this, and, as previously discussed, when parents assume the role of teacher, it can get in the way of the most important thing for their child's self-esteem, which is the relationship between the two of them.

So as a good-enough parent, find the sweet spot where you are offering support to your child on what they are learning in school, support them to do the homework as much as they can and read with them in a fun and relaxed way, but don't get sucked into a stress vortex, feeling you need to revolve your whole life around their education or their so-called deficit. As with so many aspects of parenting, it is about finding the balance between, on the one hand, avoiding or ignoring the problems, or on the other over-investing and trying to find a perfect solution. The former means your child doesn't get any help; the latter can mean they end up problem-saturated, with their life organised by what they are less good at.

WHAT DOES THE GOOD-ENOUGH PARENT DO ABOUT PRIMARY EDUCATION, THEN?

In a good-enough environment, natural ability will find its own resting place. Your kid will have inherited all sorts of abilities and possibly disabilities from both their genetics and their unique make-up. Some will be naturally academic, musical, artistic, sporty or entrepreneurial. Some less so.

In the context of the do-better-and-get-more society, the move from an education to a qualifications system and the glorification of busyness, kids can get sent off on a trajectory where they become hooked on praise or, conversely, feel like they have permanent disabilities, whereas they just have a faster or slower learning profile. The belief that it is *all* down to individual effort has become an arms race of hard work, doing more and more, whilst breaking the mental health of many of our young people and disenfranchising many others. Some of it is also about a different developmental trajectory, time and age – kids catch up; or they don't . . . But they can still have a good-enough life.

Think carefully about your child's school, obviously, but don't get too swayed by it being, on paper, a 'good' school. A madness around 'good' schools has infiltrated society, based on exam results (like the SATs), spurious inspections and reputation. It impacts the housing market, for example, which leaves us parents literally over-invested in our children's future achievement with a huge mortgage.

What does a 'good school' actually mean? It's a difficult question, but it is certainly more than test or exam results. When I was a governor at my children's primary school, part of my duties was to look at and analyse those SATs in detail. One of the years I was doing that, the school was one of the top performing schools in the whole country – if you had googled 'best primary school in the UK' or something like that, this school would have been in the top ten. But I knew the children in the school: we were top that year because of the particular children in that year; we definitely weren't going to be the following year, as we had a different group of children: bright, sparky, funny children, but ones who weren't going to do so well on SATs. Nothing else would change: the Year 6 teacher was the same each year, and she was wonderful and inspiring, and got the best out of all her pupils. It was, actually, a very good school, not because of the results they got that one year but because they worked hard with all pupils. If there were problems, they identified them early and gave kids masses of support. But you can't make kids perform at an average level if they're intrinsically way below average. In fact, I thought it was a great school because it was largely a happy place to be – with a good leadership team, supporting their teachers, fun and enthusiastic and with a broad curriculum inclusive of sport, music, art, dance, drama, friendships, community and the children's emotional lives.

So a good-enough parent does not get too caught up in the vagaries of league tables and test scores when picking a school. You want one that has a broad curriculum, rather than one that is so swayed by the SATs or other outcomes that it over-focuses on a smaller area of learning. In my opinion, the most important thing is that your child is happy at school. A happy, unpressured childhood provides good roots for meeting our manifesto aims, as well as future success. Happiness in general in earlier childhood is strongly linked to academic performance at sixteen, and the mediating pathway of this relationship seems to be happiness with school.[liv] There is lots to be said for a local school: for getting your child into one they can walk to on their own and where they can meet the neighbourhood kids to ride their bikes, go to the park or easily pop to each other's houses.

Then let your school get on and teach your child with support and interest from you, but without tipping into too much involvement or interference. Maybe your parenting shouldn't be about trying to secure for them a trajectory of future success? A good-enough home environment recognises that hard work, routine, discipline and consistency are important, but so are joy, spontaneity and relationships. Your job, as a parent, is to give them a sense of fun and good memories, as well as a capacity to work hard. It isn't to ensure that they achieve the top grades at a top university. There is time for schoolwork or adult-led graded activities, such as sport or music, and there is an equal amount of time to stop working and relax – and not just as a once-a-week treat! You might, indeed, need to slightly protect and inoculate your children from the stressful messages they will receive about hard work and achievement from teachers, other parents or their peers, and you do that through your relationship with them: it is that connection that gives them self-worth and not the achievements. So it is about mostly doing the homework, but on those occasions when it becomes overwhelming or distressing, just bundling your kid into the car and going to buy ice cream, telling them, 'Babe, it's important, but it's not that important. It's not as important as you, or your happiness.'

In that way, they are learning that they can bear the perceived disappointment of the teacher or not being the top of the class. And you are teaching them the incredibly important message that they don't always have to do their best, be their best, all the time – because sometimes all of us don't and aren't. Nothing and no one can give 100 per cent, 100 per cent of the time. We are not machines: and even machines don't work at that level of perfection. But also, these are children we are talking about, and we want the childhood years to be about thriving, not just striving.

3.3
Relationships in Childhood

I'm starting this chapter with something a bit sad.

When they head off to primary school, book bag in hand and with shiny shoes, you lose them a little bit. Your child may have been in full-time childcare or at a nursery school, but when they go off to school, they will not be so closely monitored or managed, and lots will happen to them every day that you won't know about. They won't have the words or wherewithal to tell you, and no one else will notice it. This isn't just a function of the school; it's just that children start to look beyond you, beyond adults. School-age kids get more interested in other kids. They have a pull to find other little people like them, who can share their interests or hobbies. Humans, it seems, are drawn to group together in similarity.

This is the start of their path away from you. Previously, they've been carried, toddled and taken their first steps on your path, but now the path separates. Theirs is long and the distance is hazy: you have no idea which direction it is going in. Yours runs alongside and intertwines at various points for the foreseeable future, but they now have their own path. See, I told you it was going to be a bit sad.

Your relationship-based parenting will have set them up for this new path, and for the friends they make along it. Their attachment muscle has been strengthened through the warm, reciprocal time you have spent together, but also through the rupture and repair of your comings and goings through their early years. From that, they have the little nugget of warmth and love inside them, which allows them to separate from you, and gives them that good-enough feeling as they face things alone. But also, the important things they have 'learnt' from the child-led play they will now be able to use in these other relationships. The relationship between you has taught them more intrinsically about give and take, sharing and tuning in to other people more than any dictates to share or time outs for not doing so. The imprint of that relationship gives them a well of empathy inside of them to use in their play.

What they will likely be unable to do is tell you about their separate path. It seems a universal phenomenon that the answer from children of this age to the question 'What did you do at school today?' is 'Nothing'. That leads to the two aims for this relationship chapter: how you keep your relationship with them going in the childhood years and how you support their burgeoning relationships with their own friends.

KEEPING YOUR RELATIONSHIP GOING

As their path begins to veer away from yours, your relationship with them inevitably changes. In terms of our attachment dance, they are no longer always dancing with you; they are off dancing elsewhere for several hours a day. And when they come back, sometimes they want to show their moves, and sometimes they want to join in with your dancing again. But sometimes they don't: sometimes they want separation when they come back to you, to practise their new moves on their own. They want to be off away from you or with their friends elsewhere. Sometimes they need help coming back to dance with you.

As parents sucked into the busyness business of the primary-school years – rushing between the Bermuda triangle of work and home and school – time disappears. It can be hard to prioritise our relationship with them, when our whole life is busy around them. This can leave us too exhausted to properly relate, and instead, each day can become a list of instructions for them. It is also easy to hold the false illusion that all the busyness secures our relationship with them: all the money earnt, the house provided, the food bought, the meals cooked, the clothes replaced, the lifts given feel like a relationship. We are doing these things out of our love for them, I know, but they are not generally experienced as acts of love by our children. In fact, they are totally taken for granted. The unconditional giving we are doing will leave our kids as grateful as we are on a daily basis to have our utility supplies pumped into our home: i.e. not at all. Now, of course, two generations ago, my granny, I imagine, was super grateful, awe-struck almost, to get electric lights. I still remember my mum's delight at the dishwasher – she told it how much she loved it every day as she loaded it! But me, not so much. I take these things for granted. The hedonic principle is that we get used to what we have got, and take our background stuff for granted, and for our kids, our busyness sacrifices become their background expectations, and they will totally take them for granted, too. As with you and your utilities, they will only notice parenting at all when it is not there.

Finding time for connection and communication can be tough, especially with multiple children, being busy at work and their activities. But in those first years at primary school, I would encourage you to continue joining them in the child-led play, as it is a window into their lives. They won't be able to tell you what is going on for them, but you will likely see it reflected in their play, as they will often act out versions of what they experience at school, and what they are figuring out in their little heads. Playing with them, or rather letting them lead the play, is listening to them; it's the equivalent for an adult of 'let's have coffee' – it's time to catch up and reconnect. And God forbid if anything is wrong, and if they can't tell you, this is your best chance of hearing about it. Child-led play is one of children's major routes for communicating – for touching base and for you gaining insight into their world.

The free play is important, too, which as previously discussed may need a vague supervisory presence in younger years, but should become independent later on. Time to run and be wild is crucial for some children, perhaps especially the boys, who, on average, are less good at sitting still in school. It can be boring as a parent, sitting and waiting in a park whilst they run around, and you feel a sense of urgency that you are not getting things done. The busy-ness business of better and more sells a false premise – that you are only doing something if you are engaging in their formal lessons or your chores. Those things can feel like an achievement to the busy parent – they are tickable off a list. Remind yourself, then, that sitting on the edge of the park, doing your minimal supervision-thing, with them playing with their friends or kicking a ball around or doing cartwheels by themselves, is important, too. It's the same stuff that the formal classes offer – physical fitness, practice, learning, letting off steam – but with the added benefit of having some freedom and autonomy over what they do. Adult instruction does not make an activity worthwhile, and towards our manifesto aims of feeling good enough and independence this free play matters.

Like in child-led play, bedtime is another time when kids are more porous to letting the inside stuff come out, as long as you avoid this time being hijacked by the learning agenda. The aim is a warm, relaxed time, when your kids feel safe and close to you, their defences go down and their vulnerabilities are more on display. If reading out loud is a pleasure for them, by all means go for that. But if reading is painful for them, don't force them to do it now. If you are preoccupied with reading schemes and progress, bedtime can become a fraught battle. Reclaim it for your relationship with your child. Imho, you will benefit their long-term reading more by reading to them at bedtime, in a happy and enjoyable way, than by making them torturously spell out words. As we saw in the last chapter, kids who are slow at reading generally pick it up in time, but even if they are slow, it can't dominate every part of your life.

If they do start talking more openly at bedtime, it can be quite frustrating for parents. When you are keen to get on with the chores of the evening, put other kids to bed, eat your meal or relax, your child wanting to talk about their day can feel like the final straw. You were there picking them up from school, and you asked all about it then: 'What did you do in school today, darling?' ('Nothing.') 'Oh, what was for lunch?' ('Can't remember.') 'Who did you play with at lunchtime?' ('No one.') It can therefore be easy to feel that they are dragging out bedtime or 'attention seeking'.

What does attention seeking even mean in this context? They are not looking for applause or admiration. At heart, we are animals, and we seek security before we sleep. Perhaps it means they are seeking to re-establish their attachment bond, wanting that reassurance, that closeness to you before they feel safe enough to fall asleep. They want to process the stuff of the day – the good, bad or ugly – and have it right and safe in their head to allow sleep to come. It seems when they come out of school, it is all milling around inside of them but perhaps their guard is still up from the day, or perhaps they need to burn up some repressed energy. Or perhaps it is just human nature that worries come at bedtime.

With bedtime-talking, there needs, as always, to be a balance. A very routine-driven parent may be too preoccupied with their own agenda or checklist to notice or respond to the subtle cues of distress: bedtime is 7pm and lights need to be out then, so there is no time to spot or hear about the worry. On the other hand, neither do you want to open up a whole can of worms, which may make your child more upset, and delay bedtime. You require your kind-firmness to know they need their sleep, and you need your child-free time, too. Sometimes you have to listen, understand, reassure, settle them down and get out! Sometimes it may be a bigger problem and call for a longer investment of time from you, as a parent. We return to how to address their problems later in this chapter.

FUN

The busyness agenda risks stealing all the spontaneity out of life, sacrificed on the altars of routine, activity and achievement. Please remember humour and fun. There is nothing wrong with 'scheduled fun' during family set pieces – the Friday-night movie or Sunday lunch – but manifesto-wise, giving your child a capacity for joy will be helped by your own ability to embrace it in the moment. In my family, any day with snow was an excuse to go sledging on the way to school, arriving late, with apologies that it was difficult to get there on time (not really a lie . . . it *was* difficult to get there on time, as we prioritised sledging). I imagine my kids in their whole childhood may have missed a couple of hours of education because of this but we made a lifetime of memories.

So I'm not just talking about scheduled fun, or (necessarily) the expensive holiday or special day out. Indeed, there can be a pressure on those occasions because of your time and money investment, and that can lead you to being resentful when your child behaves badly. No, the fun I'm talking about is the fun of kitchen dancing, silly walks, setting off sprinklers on a sunny evening, lighting a fire on a cold day and toasting marshmallows, spontaneous dress-up sessions, having a day when you don't do anything; or letting the kids choose all the meals. This sort of fun isn't routine or outcome-based: it's silly, irreverent and upturns the rules. I still remember the bellyache laughing of my dad daring my mum to spit a cherry stone at him, and then chasing her to throw water over her in return. They were showing me that being a grown-up was going to be OK; nothing to worry about there. It wasn't just a list of chores or hard work – it also involved shrieking with laughter. One of my favourite lines about parenting, from a book called *The Idle Parent*, is 'Kids love a tipsy mum' – perhaps because when we are tipsy, we remember to be playful again.[iv] Obviously, again, balance: they don't love a regularly drunk parent. The holiday I read that book my children learnt the important life skill of making me an early-evening G&T and bringing it to me on the sun lounger. Upturning the rules of life, them feeling grown up and independent, me showing them that being an adult was fun, me feeling relaxed . . . win, win, win.

As your kids pass through primary-school years, they may develop all sorts of changing interests, from dinosaurs to Spurs or from flower fairies to Sabrina Carpenter, and you paying attention to these shows your children that they matter to you. It's being in their headspace and thinking about what they are thinking about, in the same way as child-led play. But that balance . . . as I warned in the busyness chapter, this isn't about you taking over or becoming over-invested. It's about lying on the sofa, listening, letting them be the expert on their thing, but not trying to organise and improve their way of doing it. Too much parental investment can make an interest hard to move on from, and keeps kids infantilised.

Primary-school years are some of the most rewarding for parents on the whole. Your kids generally adore you; they can't imagine being without you. They are unquestioning of your fiefdom; the hierarchy remains in place whether you commit to the relationship, commit to busy-ness, or, quite frankly, if you are neglectful. Even kids who are abused tend to love and accept their parents in these middle years. But time spent on the relationship now is setting up the invisible infrastructure not only for your relationship with them in teenage years, but also for all their future relationships. When you relate to your children, you are setting the standards and expectations by which they will unconsciously judge all other relationships. You are, for all you learning-agenda junkies, teaching them to relate.

THEIR FRIENDSHIPS

The wonderful psychologist Brené Brown talks of the difference between fitting in and belonging. Fitting in is a state where you are constantly on edge, trying to lessen the difference between yourself and other people. When they go to school, inevitably, unconsciously, children are fitting in at first. Hopefully, over time, they develop a sense of belonging within their school, teachers, class group and peers.

There are two different ways you are going to be helping them make friends. The first is by practically supporting and scaffolding the logistics of their friendships. Of course, this scaffolding was less required in days when more kids went to the local school and there was more free play outside, but nowadays it helps if you are there in the playground, meeting the other parents, grandparents, childminders or nannies, to make play-dates and connections. Knowing their classmates' names and understanding who does what – which gym or football club they all go to, for example – allows you to maximise opportunities for them to meet their friends outside school, whilst, of course, not over-scheduling them. You want your home to be somewhere nice that their friends want to go to. Infant friendships can flourish through these parental connections, and your kid will likely be more included if you are included, too. I know, this stinks for us working parents, and, indeed, for parents who have struggled with friendships themselves and aren't comfortable in this setting.

The second way of supporting their friendships is with all the relationship-based parenting you have done and continue to do. It's in these middle-childhood years that we begin to see the reverberations from the parent–child relationship in the friend–friend relationship. When a child has experienced reciprocity and synchronicity in their baby and toddler years, it provides a good foundation for friendships. In a similar way to how they have absorbed language from you, they will have internalised the give-and-take from your goo-goo-gah-gah parenting and child-led play. Whilst this is sometimes hard for them to do, when their feelings are running high, for example, you have given them the best example to learn from.

Conversely, the costs of extreme parenting may show up in playtime: the perfect parent has struggled to demonstrate a laissez-faire attitude – they have inadvertently taught by example that things need to be 'just so'. Whilst their words may have exalted the importance of 'playing nicely' with others, their child will have felt and observed something different – control, correction, rules, rigidity. Their kids have less experience from their attachment relationship of the relaxed, easy-going attitudes that make friendships flow.

Perfectionism in parents is linked to their children being insecurely attached, and, from my observations, girls who have insecure attachment may cause particular havoc in primary years.[lvi] They unconsciously play out or replicate their experience of inconsistent attachment from their early years with their parent in their school friendships, by this time being the one in charge, rather than the one who is feeling unseen. These insecure little girls are particularly fond of being a leader in a friendship trio. Having two girls competing for your goodwill or attention is a sensible (if completely unconscious) strategy if you lack internal certainty of attachment. So one day, friend A's confidences are whispered to best-friend B, B sits beside her at lunch and B is her preferred partner for PE. The next day, she shifts her focus to best-friend C. When either B or C is in the 'left-out' position, they blame themselves, constantly try to change themselves to make A like them more, to fit in with her preferences and repeatedly chase that feeling of belonging they get when they are in the best-friend position. This keeps B and C in a state of discombobulation, as they never know where they are. Plus, the competition between them prevents them from connecting to each other. It can be heartbreak for them every other day, and for the parent watching them going in like lambs to the slaughter.

This may be your daughter's sad introduction to the on-off friend. Most grown women know what an on-off friend is without further explanation; some have even admitted to being one. Whether part of a trio, a best friend duo or a leader in a group in secondary years, it can be a toxic pattern. It is good for neither the little leader unconsciously acting out her insecurity through hurting others, nor the best friends seeking security through vying for her attention. It can get played out again in romantic relationships in future life with the on-off boyfriend or girlfriend.

In primary years, there does tend to be a sex split with girls and boys playing separately. There are likely to be both nature and nurture reasons for this – kids are looking for the belonging that they hopefully had in their attachment relationship with their parents, and sometimes we seek belonging through similarity. It can be hard talking about gender, as inevitably these are typical patterns and not absolutes. Of course, many boys and girls do not fit closely to the norm, or perhaps are tomboys or tomgirls (i.e. they prefer the sociocultural accoutrements that are not typical of their own biological sex – for example, the play, clothes or company).

I think these sex differences are worth thinking about, though. Once, visiting a girls' school, I stood with the deputy head overlooking the playground. This was a girls' secondary school and their playground ran alongside a boys' one. The deputy head told me that when he looked down at the two playgrounds, he saw two different patterns: on the whole, the girls would clump together, sometimes arm in arm, talking and whispering; the boys, on the whole, would run around.

Generally, girls' play and friendship rely more on language and communication, and boys' on shared activities and games. Girls' games tend to be more imaginative, rather than the rule-bound ones that are more the preference of boys. Girls are often creating a shared mental space between them through their words. I explain this to my young patients by drawing two girls with thought bubbles appearing from each of their heads and merging. To do this, they need some degree of what we psychologists call theory of mind, which we touched on earlier (p. 100). This is the capacity to understand that other people have minds that contain different stuff from ours. They therefore explain stuff to each other, as they know what the other one does and doesn't know. They take into their minds, from an early age, the ideas, thoughts and feeling of others, and become good at predicting what they don't know.

Boys' play at this age tends to be more physical and sport-based, built on competition, rather than collaboration, and less reliant on language. They play games where there is little negotiation – the rules are set by someone else. For example, in football the rules already exist, and are not co-created as part of the play, as they are (more typically) with girls playing 'horses' or 'schools'. This can lead to boys' friendships seeming 'simpler' or less troublesome than girls'.

Researchers debate the degree to which this is innate or taught by social gender norms. Are they born like this? Or do we impose these playing styles on children through our expectations of them, our choice of toys for them, what they observe in society? As usual, the truth likely lies in the middle. It seems that sex (nature) differences get amplified by what they see and how we socialise them (nurture); children seeking belonging and acceptance with their peers comply with the gender norms they see. I think girls' participation in football in the UK vs soccer in the US is a good illustration of this. Soccer is seen as a female sport in the US, and girls' participation in it is only slightly lower than boys'.[lvii] But as female football receives more press coverage and becomes more normal in the UK, post Euros 2022, we see more girls taking part in the sport here.

But the sex differences in play reflect a pattern of relating that is relevant when we think about children's and adolescents' wellbeing. In psychology, we talk about girls internalising what is going on for them and boys externalising. Girls relate and play by taking into account the opinions of others. Boys relate and play doing things outside of themselves; they use the physiological release of physical activity. This pattern of internalisation and externalisation is reflected in how girls and boys express their difficult feelings of anger, sadness and worry. For girls, their tendency to internalise means these feelings often stay inside them; they blame themselves for not being good enough. When boys have that feeling of not being good enough, they tend to externalise it, in displays of non-compliance or aggression. That means that girls show up more frequently in CAMHS for assessment of anxiety or depression, and boys for assessment of ADHD, or later on in Youth Offending Teams. The behaviour is different; the feelings, often not so much.

My own view, based on the children and adolescents I've seen, would be that each could get something from the skills of the other. Many girls could gain from not overthinking and just taking part in active games, whilst many boys could benefit from developing an emotional language, to understand their own experience and tune in to that of others. For that reason, as a mum, I encouraged gender neutrality in play, activities, books and emotional expression – but despite that, my girl talks to me far more than my boys. Sex difference? Socialisation? Or simply a coincidence? I can remember one very sad day, when we faced a loss in our family, and I said to one of my sons, 'Do you want to talk about it?' and he said, 'That's the *last* thing I want to do.' It wasn't my proudest moment as a psychologist parent, but it also taught me an important lesson: that not everyone wants to talk about problems. Some people have different ways to deal with them.

Supporting them with friendship and other problems
They go off to school, fresh and new, and full of hope, and developmentally they are at an age when they start to want more

people than just you. Here there is an inextricable risk that they will end up getting hurt.

Of course, we hope their friendships will be full of play and fun, sharing and kindness: that people will like them, and they will belong. Or that they will make nice friends, and it will all go swimmingly. But inevitably in life, when they start to want friends and to attach to other people, hurt is a risk.

This can be a difficult time for the good-enough parent: we know consciously that we need to support their independence in friendships, but it is so darn hard. Other children being mean to our kids can bring out rage in all of us. In middle childhood, girls seem to have more friendship issues than boys. Boys do have them – there can be problems of bullying, aggression, over-competition and sometimes exclusion – but friends generally seem to be a less problematic issue for them. With girls' friendships, based as they are on shared feelings, internal stuff, it's just more personal and more upsetting, it seems.

Here is the pattern: your child comes home with a tear-stained face and tells you about the problem. You comfort her and tell her to forget about the friend in question, that they're not a proper friend, and why not try playing with someone else instead? She says that you don't understand, and finds it hard to settle to sleep, getting up with spurious worries and concerns. She goes back into the playground the next day to find it is her day 'belonging' with the on-off friend; she is in the spotlight of her friend's attention and totally ignores your advice. You probably don't realise it, as she comes home happy the next day, but the pattern will repeat a few days later, as she feels as hopeless to resist the on-off friend as a moth to a flame. A parent who values control will quickly get frustrated that their child is not doing as they are told, and the child will then stop talking about it because they are getting advice that they just can't take.

The irony is parental standards and expectations grow into our children like the rings in a tree trunk, but parental advice rarely gets taken. Here starts one of the most difficult parts of parenting: supporting someone when you don't agree with what they are doing, and you think you know best. They are on their own path now, remember, and whilst (at this age) you are still guiding their direction in many areas, in friendships you are not so much. The reality is that you probably don't know best; the school playground is a different world. And whilst giving advice and taking control are very tempting, they can lead you to the equally unhelpful places of either being dismissive or emotionally over-involved. These are the two ends of our good-enough continuum in a slightly different form: we can shut down conversations because they don't take our advice anyway, and we are busy and tired; or, incensed by stories of unkindness towards our child, we want to storm in, guns blazing. It can be hard to tolerate that middle position of listening and understanding.

Be wary about intervening, however incensed you feel. Indeed, being incensed is probably a red flag that you shouldn't intervene. Of course, if consistently, a child's stories reflect systematic bullying over time, a parent needs to contact the school, but it is also true that kids use the word 'bullying' instead of saying more accurately 'unkind to me today' – i.e. 'So-and-so was bullying me', when they mean 'So-and-so left me out/didn't want to play with me/called me something I didn't like/whispered about me'. And of course, whilst none of these is ideal, kids are unkind and thoughtless to each other a lot. They leave someone out one day or make them the butt of their jokes. Your kid will likely do it, too. You can't charge in every time, but nor should your children's feelings about this be ignored.

It is worth mentioning that intervening by contacting the other parent is rarely successful. Your respective kids have made their cases as effectively as the defence and prosecution barristers in a court of law, and parents often feel the emotion keenly. It requires the emotional intelligence of trying to understand the dynamic of the situation, rather than assigning blame. As adults, we can have lofty ideals of friendship: everyone should be included or invited, for example. Yet children want to play with children they like, and whilst it's truly heartbreaking for your child if they are left out – for you and them – you phoning their mum is unlikely to make that other kid like yours more. They are going to think your child is someone who tells adults, which is one of the worst sins in a child's eyes. You can't force a child to be friends with someone; they may end up tolerating your child more, but with the unkindness going deeper underground, which can be worse.

Mostly, children intuitively know this and don't want their parents to intervene, but sometimes they do, particularly if they are feeling victimised or aggrieved in some way. Yet friendship issues are wave-like – they come and go, and by the time you intervene they are likely in a calmer place, and will be embarrassed, and you risk making it worse. So whilst sometimes in these primary years they need you to intervene, the bar is pretty high; in most instances, the dual-wunderkinds – empathy and curiosity – are your best tools.

Empathy and curiosity are, in fact, a little bit magic. They can be the keystones to maintaining your relationship with your child and can also be your psychological first-aid kit for all the hurts, scrapes and falls from middle childhood onwards. Keep them nearby, like Savlon and Calpol. Try not to run out of them. Keep yourself well enough that you don't.

Empathy is the emotion of understanding someone else, seeing the world as they see it. Stepping into their shoes is so important when your child is experiencing the disconnection of friendship difficulties. Understanding the facts (or rather, the facts from their point of view . . .) is part of this process, but really the empathy we are looking for here is the empathy of emotion. Empathy is not wedded too strongly to the facts: children (like all of us) tell one side of the story – the one where they (we) are not culpable. And whilst you were not there, and you did not experience the event, if you listen hard enough to their story you will likely recognise the emotion from other experiences. Tapping into that emotional memory will open up a well of understanding in you.

When we are listening to their stories, we are tempted to start pointing out their culpability or trying to squeeze the learning out of the situation, teaching them right from wrong. In fact, understanding people's feelings is often a first, crucial step before we can even begin to think about our own role in it. It is only once they've experienced the empathy of your understanding that they can sometimes begin to reflect on their own role; otherwise, they will likely be defensive to your opinion. But empathy is not just understanding how they feel and communicating that you get it; it is often sitting with their feelings about it. And this is the hard bit for a parent – the bit where you are sitting in the middle, neither getting frustrated with them for not taking your advice, nor getting incensed at the other child and storming into school. One of the key skills that you may have to learn over these middle-childhood years is accepting that you can't solve all their problems neatly and quickly. You can't now, and you can't in the future. No, the empathy is being with the problem.

Curiosity is the skill you need to find the empathy. Some of the problems children and adolescents bring me in therapy, I've literally seen a thousand times before. Often, I'm pretty certain within the first ten minutes of the session where we are going to be in the last ten minutes, but them telling me about it for the middle thirty minutes is part of the process. It would be quicker, if we could miss out the middle thirty minutes, but that is not how humans work. They wouldn't know I understand – that I am committed to understanding them – and they get that by me being curious, open and asking lots of gentle questions. And to be fair, despite all my experience, sometimes I'm wrong in my assumptions: sometimes, through my curiosity, I learn something awful or sad that they've never told anyone before. Including their parents. And they haven't told anyone before because no one has really asked: by *really* asked, I mean asking with empathy, quietly, with time and being prepared to hear.

The curiosity we are looking for is gentle, patient and gives space. It is not intrusive; this is not an inquisition. There may be silences. It looks like checking back in that you have understood: 'So was it like this? Or like that?' It might look like offering some emotion words to capture their feelings: 'Were you disappointed/frustrated/aggrieved?' It might mean making links with something that has happened before or an example from your own life when you think you felt similar: 'Was it like that time . . .?' Curiosity also requires that you let go of knowing best or knowing them best; it allows you to see the world through their eyes. It shows an acceptance for them to change and grow, without doing that thing that parents are wont to do when they characterise and crystallise their children's personality from about seven years old and define them like this.

Now, you may disagree with me on the causes of the adolescent mental-health crisis. You may not see that parenting and education in childhood are contributory factors. You may believe that it is all down to social media and to young people being snowflakes. That nobody talked to you in this way when you were a kid and you were fine. But times have changed. Whatever the causes of the mental-health crisis, I would argue that in our fast-paced, global, social-media driven world, this sort of talking gives kids the skills to navigate it. It gives them the sense of mattering to someone, of being valued. It helps them to develop the emotional insight necessary to cope with both the 500 TikToks a day they'll watch in their teenage years and an uber-competitive education system.[24]

Using empathy and curiosity helps children to think through the options and encourages their independence without negating their feelings. It helps them to solve the problem for themselves, and improves their emotional competence at naming the tricky dilemmas in life. Most of what I do in therapy comes down to these two things. If you are picking up this book for the first time in middle childhood, and have regrets, empathy and curiosity can be hugely restorative and reparative to your attachment with your child, and through this to all their future relationships.

Facilitating them to solve their own problems, with empathy and curiosity, might sound something like this: 'Gosh, that sounds really hard, what could you do? . . . Well, yes, I could contact their mum, but if she tells them off, do you think that is going to help? I think that might make them a bit mad at you. What other options have we got? Yes, it is horrible when she does this on-off thing . . . But I'm not sure talking to her

---

24 Estimates vary but lots of young people are on TikTok two hours a day; 500 TikToks is a guestimate based on this amount of use and on every TikTok being fifteen seconds long. Of course, some are much longer, but many they scroll past in three seconds.

mum will make it change. I wonder if she likes having you and Priya as two best friends who she plays with, then leaves out. If you think that she is always going to be like this, what could you do? What do you want to do?' By verbalising the process in this sort of way, but obviously in your own words and style, you are teaching them, by example, emotional competence. In the same way that we tend to verbalise any important skill when we are learning it – 'handbrake off, clutch down, change gear' – you are verbalising naming emotions, problem solving, etc. Gently pointing out the dilemmas, rather than giving the false hope that you can change other people, is also an important life lesson. This is nearly all empathy and curiosity, but occasionally throwing in a pinch of psychological knowledge about the way people are. Knowledge is different from advice. Knowledge is power: understanding on-off friends can be upsetting but gives your child the option to protect themselves. Like the emperor's new clothes, a lot can be gained by pointing out what is going on.

Naming their feelings is the first step to taming them. I think an emotion wheel stuck on the fridge can be a helpful addition to family life for these sorts of conversations. An emotion wheel starts in the centre with the big, catch-all emotions (angry, anxious, happy, surprised, sad) and moves out in two more layers to the more nuanced feelings (for example, hopeful, regretful or content). It helps children to develop emotional competence – because the first step to emotional competence is learning to recognise and label your feelings. And a sub-advantage for you outcome-focused parents is that they'll learn lots of new words for their English essays![25]

---

25 Emotion wheels can be found online, but the best one(!) is in my book *The You Don't Understand Me Journal.*

Empathy and curiosity are the epitome of the kindness we are looking for but remember that they don't negate firm. 'I get how you feel, and I feel for you my love, I truly do. But I still am saying we need to do this/you still need to go to school tomorrow. I know you don't like it, I know it is hard, and I will be here to support you. I know you are mad at me about it, but it is still what we are doing.'

Our relationship job in these middle years is to support them on their new, separate path. It is not to jump on that path to take over, even though we may want to. Often by this stage, our identity is so tied up with being a parent, we are tied to the idea that they need us, rather than cognisant that we are guiding them towards independence. We might like the version of ourselves that is omnipotent for our children: it increases our sense of importance and value.

As babies and toddlers, they have learnt about relationships by developing their core attachments; in middle childhood they need to start to use these as a blueprint and springboard to develop new friendships. Your job has been giving them the relationship-based, internal infrastructure to navigate this, and now you're in the pit lane to support them. You can listen, understand, nurture and guide these relationships now, but ultimately they are not under your control.

3.4
Screens, the Internet and Phones

When I thought about how firm and kind play out in this middle-childhood period, there were lots of things I could have written about. Bedtime, for example, or table manners, or simply getting them to put their bloody shoes on. Middle childhood, it seems, is one long list of telling kids what to do. But, of course, the great behaviour-management debate of the last, current and probably the next generation is that behemoth of the internet and screens. A poisoned chalice of issues for parents: whether to give them a tablet, to allow them to be on your phone on a boring journey, to buy a PS4 or other gaming console. Then the million-dollar question: when to get them their own mobile phone?

Internet and screens are arguably a tougher behaviour-management challenge for parents than any other in history. In some ways, this makes them a good example of how the principles of firm and kind play out: we can learn from screens and apply our learning to the other (easier) issues we face. But there are also some unique aspects of screens, which are less relevant to other behaviour-management situations a parent faces. The recency and scale of the digital takeover means we are playing catch-up on what these are. It is an omnipresence, the backdrop to children's lives, at school, home and for leisure. We don't know about the long-term consequences of these changes on all of us, partly because in research terms it hasn't been long-term yet.

When I see parents and children in clinic and ask them what their problems are, parents usually mention screen use in some form; but I cannot think of a single child or adolescent who has come to me and said, 'I'm worried about my screen use'. However, over the following weeks and months in therapy, it often emerges that their screen or phone use has played into or exacerbated the problems they face. I try to explain to them that when it comes to internet use, we adults are in uncharted waters. I expect that they will parent their kids very differently and look back in horror at what we did, in much the same way we think about kids going up chimneys or the cane being used in schools.

The informed parent is aware that there is considerable debate about whether screens, the internet and phones are having a negative impact on our kids.[lviii, lix] And whilst there are some differences between research studies, news headlines love to amplify these to make for contentious stories. In fact, most researchers conclude that there is a need for parents to be actively engaging with this issue with their kids, and that providers need to think more about protection.[lx] In the UK, the Online Safety Act was passed by government in 2023, and we are now waiting for full implementation. Some say it doesn't go far enough, and the rate of change online outpaces the slow wheels of government.

But this chapter is not about legislative issues; it is about how the firm-and-kind parent can parent now. In this chapter, in the childhood section, I'm mainly focusing on the generic problems with screen use at any age and then on particular issues that I think a parent needs to be wary of in childhood – those of gaming (obviously), porn (sadly) and the beginnings of phone use. In the adolescent section, we will return to look at social media, how it adds another hyper-level to the standards and expectations that are piled on adolescents, in a super-addictive form.

The dilemmas are what? Well, on the one hand, we are aware of the negative press and emerging data that screens, the internet and phones aren't good for kids. Even without the research, something about it doesn't sit right with us, as parents. It's sometimes hard to put your finger on it, but their obsession with screens, their zoned-out eyes, their lack of movement or engagement in anything else. We don't want this for our children; we should be firm . . .

But on the other hand, we have to parent in the context of the pressures on us and the cultural zeitgeist. My granny had to put her kids in a tea chest when she sorted eggs on their farm during the war. So is a screen really that bad? We need to work, often long hours in competitive job markets, to afford hiked-up housing prices, possibly commuting miles. Sometimes we just (feel as though we) need our kids to be on the iPad to give ourselves five minutes' peace whilst we send that last email. We also want our kids to be included with their friends and classmates and are aware that means having the social currency of, say, *Minecraft*. I still remember the name of the girl in my school who, shockingly, *didn't have a TV*. And how much of a social outcast I felt in school in 1982 the morning after I missed the first episode of *Fame*. We don't want our children to be left out; we should be kind . . .

When we do choose firm, it is hard to implement. Like the smartphone, my eldest was born in 2000, which makes him a true digital native, now graduated in Computer Science and working as a software engineer in the financial tech sector. You met him before, earlier in this book, and you will remember he was 'somewhat determined' as a toddler, and this continued through his childhood. I credit his success in computing in part to his having to get around any parental controls I tried to apply on successive devices and the home Wi-Fi. Actually, I suspect he saw it as sport, a somewhat irritating interruption to his gaming, but ultimately inconsequential. I, an immigrant to the digital world, was never going to win against this techie whizz-kid, although I went grey trying. It was sometimes not pretty.

Nevertheless, and despite my own failings, I vote firm on this one, particularly as your child sets out with screens. As you know, I generally vote kind when the two clash, but the unique challenges of the phone and screen need a firmer hand. Kind-firm, of course, but definitely firm. Let me tell you why.

THE CASE FOR FIRM
As the research debate trundles on, I am more convinced by the evidence 'against' screen use than that 'for' it. This is primarily because the case for screen use isn't really pro-screens at all: it is largely saying that the evidence against screen use isn't very strong. Conducting quality studies on the long-term effects of screen use is complicated by a number of factors, including the need for parents and children to adhere to strict research requirements for prolonged periods and the multiple, very different ways the internet is used. Thus, much of the evidence against is largely correlational and shows marginal average effects. This is considered poor-quality research by scientific standards. And yet, even the most ardent proponents of the risks-of-screens-are-overstated argument argue for moderation and parental involvement. For example, Oxford professor Andrew Przybylski, who seems generally of this mindset, suggests there is a tipping point in daily screen use (around two

hours a day for gaming and social media[26]) where it becomes associated with negative wellbeing.[lxi] By the time your child enters teenage years, you would have to be working pretty hard on firm, I think, to keep their use down to this; whilst accurate statistics are hard to obtain, screen use is generally estimated to be much more than this.[lxii, lxiii]

I view this research debate with slightly detached curiosity. I am wary of making screens the scapegoat for all the problems of modern youth. I think that we – parents, schools, society – love to blame the screen for all the issues today's children have. We love to because then we are not culpable for how distressed the current generation of young people are: we can maintain our perfect-parent identities whilst citing the screen as the root of all evil. But reading the source research I am convinced that screens *can* have a negative impact on *some* children; a negative impact that acts in combination with other changes we have seen in parenting, schools and society as a whole, such as the veneration of hard work, the constant pressure to do better and get more and the creep of perfectionistic standards. Yet for some young people, I'm sure screens are also a vital lifeline to like-minded friends outside of their immediate vicinity. It's complicated. We look for black and white causal relationships – the screen causes mental-health problems – whereas actually, this is perfect-storm territory, where a variety of different factors have come together to impact mental health.

Asking whether screens are harmful to children or not is, in some ways, like asking if the whole world is harmful to children – because as soon as you connect that screen to the internet that, ultimately, is what it is, isn't it? It is the world

---

26 For social media and gaming. If video/TV watching is included it is nearer 4 hours.

streamed right into your front room for your child to peruse with a simple click. When you give your child a screen, if you are not channelling firm, you are giving them access to the whole world and, perhaps more concerning, the whole world access to them. Certainly, there is wonderful, creative, connective and funny content out there, but there are paedophiles, too, and everything in between. Of course, it is different if you are giving them a screen that isn't attached to the internet, but, as you will see in Table 2 on the next page, offline screen time can still come with difficulties.

Values-based firmness

Generally, as parents, we edit and curate the world for our kids. We show them what we want them to see and mediate that through our own prisms. When we take them on holiday, we want to show them the glossy, happy bits, not the war-torn, troubled bits. When we parent our kids in the real world, we try to instil in them a sense of our values of right or wrong. But when we use screens, whether as a babysitter, a playmate, an educator or an entertainer, we risk not mediating or curating the content enough. And in so doing, I think we allow others to set the values.

Generally, values can be the antidote to outcome-based parenting because they are about the way you want to live your life, rather than where you want to get to. As a good-enough parent, you want to guide your children according to your own values, and therefore they can be helpful in thinking about the issues of screen use. There's a whole world of stuff out there on the internet, and, just like in the real world, you want to ensure their internet world reflects your values.

Values are about the sort of childhood you want them to have. Do you want to show them adventure? Responsibility?

Fun? Freedom? Or are hard work, faith, relaxation most important to you? What about family? Community? Environmentalism? Compassion? You'll find a list of values below. These are not all ones that I hold by and many of them are not in accordance with the messages of this book – the values of this book are balance (good enough), connection (relationship), boundaries (firm) and kindness; rather, they are values commonly identified by psychologists and those that I see reflected in my clinics.

Once you have a sense of the values you want to guide your parenting, think about how you demonstrate them in everyday life. How do you show them with your own screen use? For example, if I value relationship, what should that mean for my screen use when my children come into the room? Or at mealtimes? How would I demonstrate balance with screen use, as that is an important value to me? All through this middle-childhood period you want to be thinking about how you guide your child's screen use towards your values.

Table 2: Values list[lxiv]

Which values do you want to guide your parenting? It is impossible to hold too many in mind at any one time, so which five or six are most important to you?

Academic achievement		Admiration	
Adventure		Ambition	
Authenticity		Balance	
Belonging		Boundaries	
Career		Caring/self-care	
Compassion		Competition	
Confidence		Connection	
Contentment		Control	
Creativity		Curiosity	

Diversity		Environment	
Equality		Excellence	
Faith		Family	
Financial stability		Freedom	
Friendship		Fun	
Gratitude		Hard work	
Health and Fitness		Home	
Honesty		Hope	
Humour		Inclusion	
Independence		Industry	
Integrity		Intimacy	
Joy		Kindness	
Leisure		Love	
Making a difference		Mindfulness	
Nature		Openness	
Optimism		Order	
Peace		Persistence and commitment	
Power		Pride	
Relaxation		Responsibility	
Risk taking		Safety	
Self-discipline		Sportsmanship	
Success		Success	
Trustworthy		Uniqueness	
Work/life balance			

SCREENS – A UNIQUE CHALLENGE?

When we last talked about firm and kind it was in the context of the toddler and pre-school temper tantrums. We saw how different parenting factions could take either concept to the extreme and how finding balance in the middle was probably the way to go. How does this balance work in middle childhood vis-à-vis screens and, by extension, more generally, with childhood behaviour?

My generation of parents was the first to have to deal with screens, and I think it is fair to say that we did so effectively blindfold. We were in a foreign country – a new digital world, where we didn't speak the language or understand the issues – we had little guidance, and only our instincts to go by. We were likely too lax. We didn't understand the risks of this new world – no one did – but the tide is turning. Social psychologist Jonathan Haidt's book, *The Anxious Generation*, has been key in this, and now we are seeing daily debates about the issues of screen use in the media, the government is trying to implement legislation, schools are looking at regulation and parents are being encouraged to take a firm stand.[lxv]

But how *do* we do take a firm stand? Managing children's behaviour, whether it's getting them to bed or out of the house, is a constantly moving situation with multiple levels of meaning, but if I were writing about these things, my advice would be similar to that in the earlier chapters: firmish and kind. But these screens, attached to the internet or not, are pesky, complex beasts. Screen use is perhaps the Everest of child behaviour management: the peak challenge to your parenting muscles. In the table below I have pulled together from research and my own observations on screens and the internet what I think are the potential risks to children and make them uniquely difficult for parents to manage.[27]

Table 3: Unique challenges of screens and the internet for parents to manage

Issue	Risk
Time spent digitally	Children spending long hours on screens will miss out on doing other stuff that's good for mental health, including sleeping, eating well, moving and being outside, connection in real life and play.[lxvi]

---

27 Where these are evidence based, I have referenced the research. Non-referenced items are from my own observations.

Content of screen use	They can see content that will be distressing to them or will change their behaviour – for example, research indicates that viewing 'perfect' bodies breeds body dissatisfaction, whilst aggressive content increases aggression.[lxvii, lxviii]
Pace of content	Faster pacing, even on shows such as *Sesame Street*, can lead to habituation to shorter attention spans, and there are links to ADHD.[lxix, lxx]
Amount of content	Clinical and personal experience point towards feeling 'wired' (overstimulated or over-wrought) by an amount of content our brains are not evolved to absorb.
Confusion with play	Gaming could be considered a type of play and is used similarly – for example, for downtime outside of work – but can lack many of the benefits of play, including safe exploration, connection and physical activity.[lxxi]
Disconnection	Screen use is often solitary, and without parents' involvement it can lead children to watch or do things that are more extreme and/or distressing.
Attraction to screen	The business model of digital content is that it is designed to be very appealing. Screens are magnetic to children.
Addiction	Gaming disorder has now been flagged within the addiction category by disease classification systems.[lxxii]
Stickiness	Whilst most children avoid the seriousness of addiction, screens do keep children hooked into wanting more and more. It is hard to move them off.
Creepage	It is easy to slip into more time and more extreme screen use.
Boredom/ default option	Screens are very low effort. Other downtime options come to feel like more effort. We lose the art of boredom.

GENERIC ISSUES OF BEHAVIOUR MANAGEMENT

The challenges of screens are new, but fundamentally the ways we have to parent are much the same as they ever were. As with toddlers: do we go down a behaviourism route, focusing on clear boundaries, following through, routine and punishment? Or do we head for gentle parenting, explaining everything and listening intently? Or do we aim for somewhere in between? In this section, I will go through the tools we have for managing children's behaviour, be the issue screens or otherwise, and indeed many of these are relevant at any age – toddlers, pre-schoolers, tweens and teenagers.

Relationship and praise
Any flavour of parenting guru is going to tell you to do the good stuff: they are going to tell you behaviour management starts with putting the time into the relationship; and they will tell you to play and to praise. They will say that any child who doesn't get attention for positive behaviour will instead seek it through negative. We've had chapters on play and relationships and these are the foundation on which behaviour management is built.

Praise? Praise is a trickier one. Of course you should praise your children; praise is important in helping to guide them as to the type of behaviour you want to see. I have two reservations, though: firstly, as with any resource, the more we have, the less we value it. If you praise your children ad infinitum, it will become just background noise. Secondly, praise can attach kids to an outcome-based childhood, whereby their performance and achievements are always being graded, so keeping them tied into the opinions of others. Praise, like salt in cooking, should be used enough but not too much. And no, I can't tell you exactly how much and when. You will have to figure that out for yourself. You probably know whether you praise too much or too little and what you need to do about that.

Boundaries and rules

Setting rules, boundaries and routines with your children is a good idea because otherwise you can end up negotiating the minutiae with them every day. But rules, boundaries and routines don't just keep parents sane – they are also important to kids, as they help them feel contained. Containment is a place of psychological and physical safety where we are free to be who we want to be because we know that someone else is taking care of things and won't let them get out of control. Containment is like going to a well-established theme park, and trusting that the bolts are all tight and the rides meet regulation standards, which will allow us to relax and have fun. Similarly, rules, boundaries and routines provide psychologically contained environments, where kids can thrive, and then, as they grow up, they push at your boundaries to discover their own. I talk a lot about the deleterious impact of outcome-based expectations in this book, how the expectations we have on our kids can spiral out of control. But that is not to imply that we shouldn't have any rules or boundaries on behaviour.

Have you ever sat on the floor in a playgroup with a toddler? They push off from you and go and explore, and then something goes a tiny bit wrong – they bump into something, or someone else has the toy they want – and they toddle back to you as their secure base. It is a metaphor for the whole of childhood. Your relationship gives the world a structure, making it a place they can approach with equanimity and not panic. There is security in routine and consistency from which children feel safe to explore.

Now, obviously, some parents love a rule and a bit of containment, and others are more laid back – and with most issues of childhood I would say as long as it's not extreme, that's probably good enough. But with screens, it's different; screens are so magnetic and sticky (see table 3, pp. 186–7) that without rules your child will likely be drawn to them too much. However laid back you are as a parent generally, setting up rules for screen use is likely to be imperative.

Compliance

Once the rules and routines are in place for our children, the issue of compliance emerges. As parents, we want our children to comply as readily as Pavlov's dogs: automatically and instinctively, without question or thought. In having children, we seem to cross a Rubicon into a belief system whereby our children should do what we say all the time, even though we know that most don't, and we ourselves may not have done so. If we hold this belief too tightly or too personally, it evokes anger. This is one of the biggest issues of middle childhood, generally and with screens in particular: the frustration of children not doing what they are told.

One of the reasons why compliance is difficult for children is because they live much more in the present; this is their charm, as well as our frustration. The organising and planning parts of their brains are not fully developed, and so their cognitive function ('this is the right thing to do') is not mature enough to override their emotions ('this is what I want to do right now'). They cannot foresee outcomes as we can, be they short-term, like making us late for something, or the long-term harm of screens. But indeed, we often forget that all of us are bad at caring about future consequences when we are engaged in something absorbing. Just think how often your desire to do something overrides your good sense: scrolling late at night? Another episode of that box set that makes you late to bed? That extra biscuit? In these moments you allow your emotions to cloud your judgment, and it is unrealistic to expect that your children will be different. So if your child is rude or non-compliant, it can be worth bearing in mind how it feels having your own will thwarted; how resentful you are when you are absorbed in your own stuff, and someone comes along and imposes their demands on you. ('What now? You want lunch? Oh, for God's sake . . . I have a book to write.')

Compliance is valued highly by adults as it makes our lives easier, but there are disadvantages of instinctive compliance, too. In my opinion, some children (often girls) comply too much. They have a fear of conflict or not following the rules. They can be left unconfident in adolescent and early adult life, perhaps putting up with stuff that they shouldn't because they have been trained to comply – things like a bullying boss or someone wanting sex with them. I have seen too many people-pleasing girls who have not left a sexual situation when they should have as it would have been 'awkward' or 'difficult'. These girls are often hooked on the good opinion of others, seeking the high of praise. So it turns out we don't want Pavlovian dogs; we don't want to squash out of kids their capacity to argue back and say 'no'.

At the other end of the behavioural spectrum, some kids will always rebel, and with them, the risk is that they will drive you into being unkind, with spirals of punishment and consequence, as we saw earlier with children placed in closets and spanked if they didn't comply with time out.[28]

As far as I can tell, throughout time, parents have always expected but not got compliance . . . and then we come to screens. With screens, we find a massive, multi-trillion-pound industry, completely dedicated to making them as appealing

---

28 We will return to these different sorts of kids in the adolescent section.

and as addictive as possible, effectively acting in direct opposition to a child complying. We are pitting all those brains and technology against the delayed gratification and willpower of a child. It makes me think of the experiment where four-year-olds were given a marshmallow and told that they could have two if they managed not to eat it for fifteen minutes. Doesn't a marshmallow seem a quaint temptation now? What sort of temptation is that compared to *Mario Kart*?

With this fateful combination of children's low compliance and screens' high stickiness it can mean that as a parent you end up at best repeating yourself, probably nagging, or, at worst, shouting to enforce screen rules. Of these, repeating yourself calmly and waiting is likely best for manifesto aims, but hard to do, especially if you hold the unrealistic belief that children should automatically comply, because that belief can make you rageful. Most good-enough parents probably end up shouting sometimes, but rageful shouting isn't great for kids, tbh. A louder, firmer voice for emphasis, whilst you are still in control, is better.

If these don't work, you may need to use consequences or punishments to get them to care more about what you are saying. Logical consequences on screens would mean turning them or the Wi-Fi off or taking the device away. They are generally most successful, as they make intuitive sense, so that kids don't get into the defensiveness of 'it's not fair'. If you can keep in mind that it's not personal, it may help you stay calm: it's not that your kid is the worst, nor are you a bad parent. Rather, it's that non-compliance is relatively normal in children and screens are incredibly hard to get off of.

The struggle is how to be firm enough but with a gentle, open tone that allows for you and your children to be on the same side: that balance to be found between firm and kind. You're not looking for sledgehammer firm because that can lead to a sense of them against you, which is counterproductive. By sledgehammer firm I mean an attitude characterised by punishment or anger, or non-negotiable, dictatorial blanket bans. Your child *will* break whatever screen rules you set because their willpower and self-discipline are no match for the addictive qualities designed into the devices. That is a David-and-Goliath fight your child is not going to win. But if you are angry, shouty and draconian about any sort of rule breaking, you risk losing all co-operation, creating a battle atmosphere of move and counter-move over where the iPad is and what the passcode is (seven failed attempts later, they work out it's the dog's birthday). This risks sending the behaviour underground or pushing them into outright rebellion, and then you will miss opportunities to teach and guide and, later on, they will not come to talk to you when problems arise.

Children also instinctively know that rules and routines change as they grow up and they will push, whine and nag to get those changes happening quicker. As they become more independent from you, they will go into other people's homes and see things are done differently and begin to question the status quo at home. This is a good thing... in theory – a good-enough parent doesn't assume that their children will be just like them and wants them to have their own thoughts and ideas. However, whilst children's pushing is important for independence, it is a nightmare for policing screen use. It would be simple if we could set a screen rule when they are six years old and it stays the same when they are sixteen. The key issue is how to be consistent, yet flexible; adjusting the rules as they get older, whilst our values remain constant.

The dilemma at the heart of behaviour management is to raise children with a strong sense of attachment; they need to know you will always be there for them and that means they can take you entirely for granted. 'Always being there' and 'being taken for granted' are two sides of the same coin. Having kids push against your authority and being ignored is super-annoying, and yet it is also a side effect of loving them unconditionally and securely. This is why children behave worse for you than anyone else: they trust your love more.

But it seems to me there are two speeds on compliance: immediate and forever. Children may or may not do as you tell them in the next five minutes, and that is frustrating, but step away from the immediate situation, and remember where the power of your influence lies. It does not lie in their momentary compliance, when they are being guided by their emotions, but in the values they see you demonstrate and the example you set. Those will become embedded in them over years, and they may choose to live by them or react against them, but, when they are adults, they will not be insignificant to them. There is no 'perfect response' you can give that will guarantee immediate behavioural compliance, I'm afraid, but your reaction will be instilled in them as a norm for their emotions, behaviour, relationships and thinking in all sorts of unpredictable ways in the future. Sometimes regrettably, our parents' opinions live on in our heads throughout our lives.

Parental attention, connection and scaffolding
Children are really attracted to their screens, and when they get on them are happy to stay on them. When we are busy – and I know you are all busy, as busyness, as we've seen, is the drug of this age – we run the risk of a habit being set up where the screen becomes the default option, whereas what we want is that the screen is just one of many things that they enjoy doing, including, as they get older, entertaining themselves. Like sugar,

they will likely want it more than is good for them. And as with food, it can feel easier to go to extremes: either firm (no gaming, no TV, no tablet) or lax (have it whenever you want). Is there a middle sweet spot where they have some screen time (so you get your peace, they know the social currency at school) but they are not on it all of the darn time?

We expect them to be able to entertain themselves as we get on with other things, even though the busyness agenda has not encouraged that independence. The screen is an easy out for us parents: it's the equivalent of feeding them pizza and chips; we will get no complaints and, jeez, sometimes good-enough parents feel like they need this. However, research with toddlers has shown that giving the screen more at three years old results in more tantrums at four years old, with cycles set up where the screen acts like a digital pacifier.[lxxiii] We make a rod for our own backs, because then getting them off the blooming thing for bedtime, to go outside and move, to eat right and connect, requires more effort from us. The tricky thing for parents is 'no, I'm not going to play or talk with you', but also, 'no I'm not going to give you the screen'. If we do this, they are going to whine, be bored, protest more, interrupt more and argue with their siblings. They are more likely to have accidents as they get into more non-screen adventures.

So as parents, then, we sometimes love the screen because when our children connect to it, they disconnect from us and we get five minutes' peace. On days when the whole parenting balancing act has worn us down, the screen can provide a solution. But I want to point out that a child watching something or playing a game alone is a very different experience for them than watching or playing something with someone else. The latter creates a sense of connection between you, and can, as they get older, allow for tricky discussions to take place about social and emotional things, which might otherwise be too intense. Which isn't to say that you have to always watch things together or do things with them: you only need to be good enough, remember.

With screens, and really most aspects of children's discipline, what we want to develop is an attitude of supportive scaffolding towards independence. You want them to be making sensible choices for themselves later on, but to do that, you will need, over the years, to show them, talk to them, demonstrate and stay involved before they get to a point where they are doing this on their own. As with food, there are temptations that are bad for them – they are going to need your guidance about their consumption of both chocolate chip cookies and *Fortnite*.

In this way, you are looking downstream to your future adolescent and shaping your child towards this. Mostly, the behavioural strategies of firmness, consequences and compliance are going to become obsolete tools in the future – they just don't work on most teenagers. Adolescents require a feeling of co-operation and respect, and telling them what to do tends to be less successful.[lxxiv] Don't underestimate the power of your own example on screens either – research has shown that to be important.[lxxv] So for now, it's about firmness, but with one eye on the autonomy that they are going to have with their screens in years to come. Discipline should be used as a path to autonomy.

Over the childhood years and into adolescence, you need to try to keep in mind that phones and screens should ideally be something you are talking about and sharing with your child, not an area of constant tension. As a firm-and-kind parent you are looking for open communication and not a fight. Of course, as you are likely only good enough, you will not always get it right, and you may get cross and frustrated, and then have to try again to find the messy middle, which is neither threatening blanket bans of all screens for ever, nor letting your children have them constantly. It is in these difficult discussions that children's emotional competence takes root.

GAMING

One of the tricky things about gaming is that it can creep into your life insidiously. One minute they are playing educational games on the BBC website, and you are in smug-parent mode; then they are building things on *Minecraft* (that's practically Lego – so good for hand–eye co-ordination! Perhaps they'll be an architect. Or a pilot!); but then drip, drip, drip, and they're suddenly starting with multiplayer Minecraft, begging you for a PS4 or Xbox and, before you know it, they're playing multiplayer shooter games. Those educational games are like cannabis: an entry-level drug.

Because, like drugs and alcohol, it seems that gaming can be addictive. Yet, also like drugs and alcohol, most people game without getting addicted, and it gives a huge amount of pleasure to a lot of people. It seems that it may only be addictive in a sub-section of society: best estimates suggest 1 per cent are addicted and a further 5 per cent have problematic use.[lxxvi] But even when kids are not addicted, it can be incredibly difficult for a parent to manage. It's what I call stickiness (see table 3, pp. 186–7). Screens, it seems, are stickier than nearly everything else, and words rarely (never?) spoken in childhood are: 'Dad, I'm going to get off this game now to do my homework or play outside.' These games are designed to keep them hooked in – they often have no natural stop.

The vast majority of researchers and clinicians now believe that exposure to violence in gaming marginally and on average increases aggression; it causes kids to be physiologically aroused, think more aggressive thoughts and behave in more aggressive ways: we know this is more of a problem for boys, not least because boys game more.[lxxvii] Violent video games also reduce prosocial feelings and behaviour, such as empathy, and desensitise young people to violence.[lxxviii] Whilst research effect sizes may be small, they will be added to those of, at best, violent films and violent music, or, at worst, violence witnessed in the home, school or community or in porn.

Long answer short, then: you are going to need firm here. Stay involved: know what they are doing, understand it, manage their access. As we've discussed, they know that as they get older, you will change the rules, and they will constantly push for more time, and for more exciting games.[29] That is very boring for you, as a parent, because you end up discussing the same thing over and over. And it's hard to find kind when you have to repeat yourself, but, of course, finding kind in the firm is always important.

So set the rules warmly and firmly in the negotiating phase. If necessary, write them down, and be clear about consequences. This sort of parenting style – authoritative, clear and kind – has been associated with mediating the negative effects of the internet.[lxxix] Both overly permissive and over-controlling parenting seem to backfire: the former because no boundaries are set, leaving a child at risk of being on screens too much; the latter, because the battle lines are drawn and children hide their screen use and are not able to talk to their parents about any screen problems they face.

---

29 That is also why behavioural theory, based on animal experiments, does not work perfectly with children: because they develop and grow, and your rules do need to change to accommodate that.

PORN AND SEXUAL CONTENT

In my work, sadly, I have often sat with people who have been sexually abused or assaulted by others. I have also sat with young people who have disclosed a history of porn exposure or use in their childhood. When the latter talk about the ways that this exposure has impacted them, it often feels as though they, too, have been abused or assaulted by this passive content. The sense of trauma and the changing of their life trajectory seems similar to that of abuse victims: of something having been done to them that can't be undone. This sense doesn't seem to be lessened even if they have clicked on it themselves. Unlike abuse victims, there is often no obvious 'perpetrator' to blame. Or, rather, who is to blame is less clear. Is it the online platforms that host this material? The government for not regulating it? Or the porn industry for luring them into ever more extreme content? And any of these might blame you, the parents, for not having appropriate controls or supervising properly. It can become pass-the-parcel on blame. This doesn't help the young people I see, and, with no one to blame, they blame themselves.

They blame themselves because porn inappropriately sexualises them when they are at an age when they can't understand it: they get feelings that they don't recognise. Curious, exciting, rebellious feelings. And so they look again, trying to understand. And again. They kind of know they shouldn't, but it's like having a sweet jar next to their bed: hard to resist, even when it makes them feel sick. Often, it changes how they relate to their peers, or how they look at other people. They get in too deep, and they don't tell because they think – they know – they would be in terrible trouble. Later, sometimes, they get into the wrong relationship, or no relationship at all. They may put themselves in real-life situations where they are abused, or they sexualise other people. Deconstructing what happens to them in therapy without shame and blame and helping them to see themselves as a victim of circumstance (for example, a lack of parental supervision, insufficient legislation or an unregulated porn industry) can help.

Recent data suggests that a quarter of children have seen porn by the age of eleven, and most have seen violent porn by the age of eighteen.[lxxx] Or, to put it another way, up to a quarter of children in the UK have been inappropriately sexualised by online porn by eleven years old. For some, it will be a one-off thing, but for others, it will be the start of their own slippery slope, as I described above. Of all the internet problems I see in my clinic, my advice to parents is more than anything, try to protect your children from porn.

How to do this is perhaps the most delicate balance of firm and kind you will ever need. Yes, get the parent controls in place for Wi-Fi and devices, but that only provides protection in your own home. The tricky bit is eliciting their own motivation not to see it. If you go sledgehammer firm, you may prompt their rebellion or curiosity, whereas you want them to be onside with you here. Children nowadays are facing a world of emotional complexity outside of strict norms or the moral code of the past, and for them to navigate it they need your guidance. That means talking to them about this stuff, probably around the time you are talking to them about sex more generally. There is no clear guidance on the best way to do this, as far as I am aware, but my instinct is to tell kids that sex is a great and wonderful thing to do at the right time, and with the right person, but that watching porn would likely ruin that experience for them. Because that is what the research tells us – that use of porn interferes with sexuality, particularly male sexuality, and affects people's expectations around sex in aggressive ways.[lxxxi, lxxxii] As a parent, I tried to explain that if they were shown porn, they could get images in their heads that might not go away and would be confusing and upsetting, and that when they did have sex these would make it less likely to be good. I remember telling one of my kids that viewing porn would be like learning to drive by watching *Top Gear*: it would give them unrealistic expectations. You also want to warn them that other people might try to show them porn, and that if this happens, you want them to talk to you about it – that you won't be cross, but it's important that they tell you.

For them to actually do this, you will need to have demonstrated in the past that you can be calm and kind about difficult things. That is why, upstream of this, when they are younger, you want to respond in a measured way to school or friendship problems. They need to trust that you can stay calm and will listen to their point of view, and if you've done that in the past it will help. They will probably fear that you will phone their friend's mum and their friend will end up hating them. If you've previously been sledgehammer firm rather than kind-firm, they will fear losing all their devices and not be open with you. To get them to talk to you about things like this, they need to feel that they have some agency in conversations with you and that you will hear them, be kind and make the right decisions.

GETTING A MOBILE PHONE

Over the last generation, the age for children getting a smartphone has consistently gone down, and now typically sits at around nine or ten. As awareness starts to increase about the hazards of smartphone use, we may be at a turning point where this age will start to rise again. Schools are taking a more active stance on banning or restricting smartphones in the classroom. A comprehensive and rather brilliant Norwegian study in 2024 showed how schools banning phones led to less bullying and fewer mental-health problems.[lxxxiii] Some schools are requesting that pupils only bring flip or burner phones, or that they lock them up for the day.

When deciding whether a child gets a phone, the issue of safety is often cited. With the disappearance of any public-phone network and kids travelling farther to school, along with the change to the active, monitoring parenting style many favour these days, it can feel 'safer' for children to have a mobile phone, so as to be in constant touch with us.[lxxxiv] Are we kidding ourselves, though? With two-fifths of crimes now involving theft of mobile phones and young people disproportionately targeted, it seems we've made kids a beacon for crime, rather than 'safer'.[lxxxv] This 'safe' feeling also ignores any psychological risks of phone use.

You will need your firm muscle to establish your values before your child gets their phone, because, from the moment they have it, your negotiating, power and influence are on diminishing returns. One thing that can be very helpful is a sense of community: one parent in one of my children's friendship groups suggested that we all get the same low-value phone. And again, some schools are beginning to facilitate this, so that groups of parents feel emboldened against the pester power of 'everyone else has got one'.[30] Nor does it have to be sledgehammer firm to decide that they are not getting a phone till later: it can be kind-firm to say, 'I hear what you are saying darling, but I am waiting another year to get you a phone. Yes, I hear that it's hard for you to be in contact with your friends without a phone, and I'm sorry. And because I know that's hard, you can use WhatsApp, Snapchat and TikTok on my iPad for an hour in the evening.'

---

30 For some examples of how schools and communities have worked together to delay children's smartphone usage, see: https://www.bbc.co.uk/news/articles/ckg2r4rxjd9o

When you are negotiating when they get a phone, it can be helpful to write down what they use it for and how much they use it in the form of a firm-but-kind contract. That is because our relationships with our mobile phones are complicated, and the psychology of this is not yet understood. It seems once we have them, we are rarely apart from them; they become almost a part of us, like an extra limb, essential to life. Do we want this for a ten- or eleven-year-old? Phones are also exquisitely private in a way that gaming and other screens may not be, and where we can see what they are up to. Writing a contract before is setting the boundaries that will structure their relationship with their phone.

That said, some phone contracts I've seen are too firm, a bit prison-guardy, too impersonal and full of unrealistic expectations, like, 'I must always have my phone charged' or, 'I must always answer promptly when my parents call'. These are absolute standards of perfection that no one can always meet. The rebellious will then use the small print of these definitive criteria to argue their case, whilst the compliant will become anxious about trying to meet impossible expectations. We're looking for something a bit more personal: a bit more kind.

I think there are three principles that are important in a phone contract: parental involvement, responsibility and values.

Parental involvement

Parental involvement is the supportive scaffolding mentioned earlier. The phone gives them access to the whole world, and the whole world access to them. You wouldn't let them wander anywhere in the world on their own, talking to whoever they pleased; you would teach them the way and guide them. Likewise, with the phone that means, especially in these younger years, looking at their browsing history in a completely upfront and open way. This isn't like reading their diary; it's supervising their exposure to all that is good and evil in the world, and it is guiding them in the same way that you would on appropriate food, clothes and handling of money. They won't make sensible choices if you leave them without guidance because they are children, and children are often daft and sometimes mean.

Responsibility

You want your child to learn that having a phone involves responsibilities – to you, to themselves and to their friends.

Their responsibility to you is your expectations around the when, where and what of phone use and charging. As I said, these expectations can be worded kindly and realistically: 'please charge your phone overnight in the kitchen', rather than 'you must always charge your phone overnight in the kitchen'.

Their responsibility to themselves is to keep themselves safe: for example, to talk to you if they are worried about something online, if someone contacts them who they don't know, if someone is mean to them or they see something they don't like or don't understand. Here, you are setting up the open communication you are expecting: 'if you are worried about something, please talk to me'. It also incorporates the responsibility of traffic and street awareness: not walking across the road with headphones in, or not looking at their phones, rather than the road.

Lastly, they have a responsibility to others: not being mean or posting stuff that will upset people. Messaging services and social media can be used to make in and out groups, which exacerbates the friendship issues we see in tweens and teens. Try to help your child see that, without falling into the trap of demonising or othering unkindness. Your kid will likely be unkind at some point, too. Almost all of us are, sometimes.

Values

This is about stating what you do and don't want the phone used for and linking these points to a general principle or specific value that both helps to reinforce what is important to you and avoids you failing to foresee every possible problem. For example, with my children, I wanted to maintain real-life times of social connection, so I banned phones in situations where we normally chatted: short car journeys and mealtimes. But you might say you want them to avoid vanity (for example, pouting) or self-obsession (for example, what they had for breakfast).

Of course, your kids will mess up. But a parent who is supportively supervising screen use will then talk to them about it and help them to understand how not to next time. In terms of manifesto aims, this is developing their emotional competence. Emotional competence doesn't believe in perfection – but it does try for an ability to self-reflect without it being a disaster, and recognising the need to apologise. Firm-and-kind parents don't rush to punish or take the phone away: they give second chances (but possibly not a third).

In my clinical work, sadly, I have seen that 'too-firm' situation playing out badly in adolescence. I see young people getting into situations with their phones that they then can't talk to their parents about, as they fear they will take them away. That leaves them on their own with the problem. That is why sledgehammer firm is counterproductive: in your move to control absolutely, your child actually ends up losing your wise counsel.

FINAL SCREEN THOUGHTS

Setting your child up well with their screen use is a challenge. The internet, gaming, phones and social media will be amongst the trickiest problems you face as a parent. You were probably not aware of that when they were toddlers and you first gave them an iPad or your phone for some peace and quiet and an easy life. In contrast, as they get older, it becomes the issue that needs more of your time, involvement and supervision than any other, especially if it goes underground or becomes a bone of contention. It is often difficult to know what to do, but the principle of firm and kind will guide you. You might also want a side order of values.

PART 4: TWEENS AND TEENS

PART 4:
TWEENS AND TEENS

4.1
The Perfect Storm – The Adolescent Years

The end of primary school and the start of secondary school has always been a significant marker in a child's development. Traditionally a time when kids start travelling further away from home alone – both metaphorically and physically. Now, also the timing of a second significant marker, where even the most intransigent parents tend to give in and allow a smartphone, and consequently play and communication move online. Whilst official teenagerdom is still a couple of years off, this is where their path takes a sharp turn away from yours. Quite simply, more of their path is out of your sight – on the bus to school, at a school where you don't know most of the pupils and parents and, of course, the weird private-exposure of the smartphone: privacy from you; exposure to the world.

SYSTEMS AND MENTAL ILL HEALTH

It is in these years that I too often see all the factors that have been bubbling away for years come to a head. We've covered so much ground in this book, so many different issues that can have an impact on a child, and here, in the adolescent years, we are in danger of all of them reaching their peak and clashing into each other in a perfect storm. There is a risk of that storm worsening mental health.

Yet, although we've covered a lot in this book, we haven't covered all the elements that impact on mental ill health. There is a considerable genetic and neurobiological component, which increases or decreases our vulnerability to mental illness in the same way that we are born with a predisposition to certain physical illnesses. Then, some kids have terrible things happen to them – some lose a parent or experience abuse, ill health, bullying. We also saw the impact of Covid on young people: how, denied the normal developmental pathways of socialising and separation, so many suffered. Mental health is a continuum, and Covid, for example, pushed many young people over the edge from just coping to not coping. Indeed, beware of anyone offering you a simple causal explanation of your or their mental health. Mental health is not simple: there is rarely one cause. An infinite number of factors make up each of our moods and mental states – many of which are not under our control

But some of them are: when you are thinking about giving your child the best chances for good mental health, you should think in terms of a biopsychosocial model. So we have their unique genetic or biological risk factors and they will also have their individual personality and psychological make-up – their thinking styles and behavioural habits, for example. But also, any young person lives in multiple systems (see diagram on next page) and these can support or undermine mental health. One of them is their family system, and that includes you, their parents.

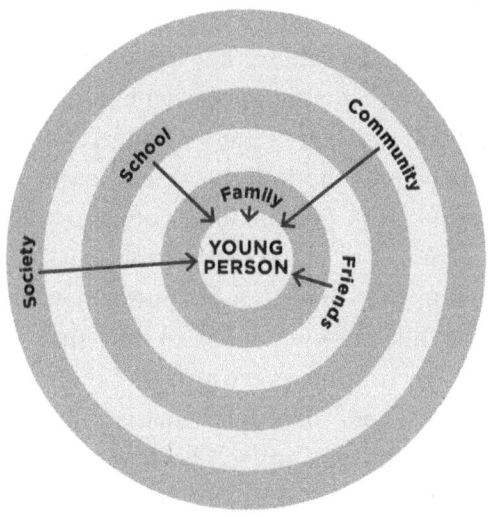

Over the thirty years I've been working as a psychologist with young people, I have noticed how systemic changes in society, communities, schools, friendships and families have acted together to worsen mental health. These changes are the ones I've been tracing in this book: ones that increase a culture of comparison, competition, getting more, doing better, expectations, striving and self-improvement.

I see this in increased globalisation, for example, where adolescents have a sense of competing on a global stage, be this online, for university places or in a global economy. I see it in our veneration of busyness, our long-work-hours culture, the idea that we need to buy more or 'better' goods and experiences. I see it in the qualification-obsessed education system – kids vying for places at 'better' schools or travelling further away from home to go to one. I see it, of course, on the internet, with adolescents constantly competing with someone on a higher level of their game, or an influencer with more followers than them, or someone working harder, or running further or looking 'better'.

It seems that when, from early in life, children are placed in lots of situations like these they often end up feeling not good enough. And feeling not good enough inevitably elicits difficult feelings: anxiety, sadness or anger. Which of these they feel depends on the individual, and each plays out in different ways. If they feel anxious, young people often end up trying to control or avoid things: this might start small, with the feeling that they should control how their school bag is packed, but often escalates to how they can control their eating, their routine, every aspect of their day. Alternatively, if they feel sad, sometimes that is unbearable – they want a way out and end up self-harming. When they feel angry, they might want to drop out or express their anger in violence against society.

We, as adults often get very preoccupied with these symptoms; these representations of the feelings. We try to treat the self-harm, eating disorder or violence. But really, we need to go to the source of the feelings and that is, often, the multi-level, implicit and explicit pressure that is coming at adolescents from all around them. A pressure that pushes some of them to run on a hamster wheel of self-improvement, towards a mythical perfection, or leads to a sense of learned helplessness, a feeling that they might as well give up, as they'll never make that (perfect) grade, so why bother, for example, going to school? And that is what we see in the research: there has been a huge increase in levels of perfectionism in Western society amongst college students, which leaves them hugely vulnerable to mental illness.[lxxxvi]

So I believe there is a perfect storm of factors that's pushing so many of our children over the line into mental ill health. It seems that in a drive to improve standards, we have shot past good enough, which promotes the relaxed, flexible environment for happy development, and instead created a storm of pressure, of extremes and of expectations on young people. I think had this been a mass societal experiment in how to raise children, we would have to say it had failed.

As I said, there are endless contributory factors to any storm of mental ill health, all overlapping and interacting, but in this chapter, we will be looking at just a few of them: the tween and teen psychology, the education system, the impact of the internet and social media and perfect parenting. Finally, we will look at how you can mitigate all this through a good-enough parenting stance.

TWEEN AND TEENAGE PSYCHOLOGY
When I see my patients and their parents to discuss their mental illness, they are often looking for fault or blame. How did this happen? The parents generally blame 'the blooming phone' and sometimes pressure from their child's school. When I give talks in schools and ask teachers about what *they* think is going on, they also tend to blame social media, but pushy parents as well. In society, politics and the media, too, there are narratives of blaming parents: either for being too involved (the so-called 'helicopter' parents) or not involved enough (not getting children into school or not keeping them off the streets). And there is also a societal narrative blaming the young people themselves – claiming that they are snowflakes, or not resilient or that sort of thing.

I see these single-cause explanations as too simplistic and multi-causal reasons as more compelling. And one of the contributory factors is the psychological stage of adolescence itself. The influential developmental psychologist Erik Erikson coined the phrase 'identity crisis' to capture the psychological task of this age. Whilst we saw how, in the baby years, babies are wired to tune in to their parents' faces to establish attachment, in the teenage years, they are wired to look away from their parents, outside of family and home, and to look instead to peers and society, moving towards separation and, ultimately, procreation. Comparing and contrasting themselves to others has always been part of this process. Nowadays, however, they do it having been compared and contrasted and engaged in multiple systems of competition and self-improvement from an early age. They do so having been trained into a comparison mindset throughout their childhood. They do it in a society hyper-tuned to comparison with league tables, 'best' listings and top tens.

So when they look outside themselves in their search for identity, they find this complex, fast-moving smorgasbord of other people's opinions and ideals. They find a societal zeitgeist of busyness, hard work and constant improvement, with shifting goal posts, where success is always over the next hill. They may have their parents exhorting them to behave, study, practise and to do their best, to eat right, exercise more, get off their phones . . . And in school, they have almost certainly been constantly marked and graded, encouraged to aim higher, to improve and improve again. And then, when they try to escape those explicit pressures for a few hours, they turn to their phones, the ubiquitous leisure activity of the day, and there they are insidiously immersed in the implicit yardsticks of the internet: often fake, usually extreme, there is always someone doing more and looking better. On every front in their search for identity they find an extremity that they cannot reach.

Adolescence has always been a difficult time. As a time of change, it can create a state of flux and insecurity in adolescents as they try to figure out who they want to be. Life is uncertain, and uncertainty is anxiety provoking. Because of this search for identity, and also the increased interest in sex, it is a time when self-consciousness peaks. The adult world, society, is meant to be a ballast to this, to keep them steady and on track, to keep some balance, as they search (or flail around) for identity. Instead, we risk adolescents finding extreme standards to live up to (or opt out of) wherever they look: from screens, from schools and, if we are not very careful, from ourselves, as parents.

THE EDUCATION PIECE

In Chapter 3.2, 'School and Education', I described how the GERM (Global Education Reform Movement) has spread to many countries of the world. The reform has noble aims to improve standards and give more kids opportunities, but often now results in schools that focus less on educating children or engaging them as useful citizens in society, and more on passing exams. But particularly in the tween and teen years, there is a move away from giving kids a broad range of experience, knowledge and skills and towards learning rote facts for a short period of time to get them over the line to the next stage of education or on to a career. Kids are taking exams to be allowed to sit other exams, where only some of the knowledge at the previous stage is built upon. It is a pyramid scheme of exclusivity, increasingly weeding out children, leaving fewer at each level up.

So sadly, many formal qualifications are not about bringing kids up to a particular standard and then giving them a qualification stating that they have met that standard – like a driving test. No, they are a system of ranking children from those who do the best to those who do the worst, allowing only some of them to progress to the next level. In the UK's GCSE exams, for example, in the top grades, there has been an arms race over the last thirty years, with governments subdividing an A grade to create an A* and then subdividing that into an 8 or 9 grade.[31] Kids who used to be thrilled with an A are now chasing an A* and end up disappointed that they can't meet this just-out-of-reach standard they were encouraged to strive for. But for the kids at the other end of the academic-achievement scale, there is an artificial boundary, below which children are said to have failed despite there being three grades below this arbitrary cut-off. For maths and English this applies to around a third of pupils. They keep the failure rate at this level in part to avoid criticism of grade inflation, but it makes a mockery of any attempts to increase standards as a nation.[32] And because maths and English are deemed so important, 'failing' at these leads to a massive closing down of life opportunities for these kids.

I believe the psychological consequences of this are far reaching in terms of adolescent mental health, but also for society as a whole. School should be about engaging kids in society, not just exams, but when a third of kids leave school with a sense of failure, we are disenfranchising them just before they are adults. Then we wonder why so many young people experience mental-health problems, or turn to crime, or don't want to do low-status work that is necessary for society to run: the inactivity rate for those aged sixteen–twenty-four is at a record 18.6 per cent.[lxxxvii] Those three grades below the 'fail' line which are rendered impotent by that boundary could instead be utilised to differentiate skill levels and focus on what children *can* do, rather than what they can't. I worry about these kids: they are called the forgotten third of education and I've written about them previously.[lxxxviii] This is incredibly sad for those children,

---

31 The A grade at GCSE was changed to an A and A* in 1994, and the A* subdivided into 8 and 9 grades in 2010.

32 Alfie Kohn is very interesting on this point. See his article from 16 June 2019 – 'Can Everyone Be Excellent?' *New York Times*.

but I believe that it puts pressure on all the children in the system because it actually makes the education system a mass competition, and whilst few people know that explicitly, everyone feels it implicitly.

Of course, competition is not bad per se. In some aspects of life it can be motivating, fun and appropriate – sport, for example. Humans naturally compete: anywhere in the world, give boys in particular a ball and watch them form teams and find a way to make a competitive game. But this is vastly different to the competition now at the heart of the education system. When a child is taking their formal exams, they are part of a system of social pressure that is all about those exams. They are in the news, they dominate school life, parents can be a bit obsessed with them and family life is organised by them. It is likely that most kids' friends are doing them at the same time, with the competition that brings over grades, next schools or colleges. The formal exams impinge on every part of life – if they are watching TV, we ask, 'Shouldn't you be studying for your test?' And if they *are* studying, they will likely be aware of whether their friends are also studying, and whether they are doing so more/less/differently. The tests, exams, qualifications are not just one part of their life but all-encompassing.

These exams are also high stakes. There are boundaries put in for supply-and-demand purposes into the 'best' next school or university. Courses set grade requirements based not on the intellectual capacity needed to complete them but because they can because of this competition to be 'the best'. Young people believe that their whole future depends on these exams; and yet we know that very little of our own life success or that of our friends actually depended directly on exam results; that most of us have zig-zag career paths; and that even if something bad happened in one exam, on one day when we were sixteen, it worked out in the end. We resat, or went in another direction or came back to it later. I know so many adults who returned to education later or changed careers mid-path. But this is not part of the narrative for adolescents.

There is this huge system of educational pressure around them; and *we personalise all that pressure on them.* We give them the message it is down to them and either how bright they are or how hard they work. And whilst it is important that kids have a growth mindset, a belief in their own agency, it is also important that they know it has limits. It is not *just* down to how hard they work because luck, timing and a whole heap of other external factors are also important. Despite knowing that grade boundaries go up and down, that teaching is variable, that exam marking is sometimes inconsistent, they believe that their success or failure shows something important about them: they believe that the subdivision of excellence on one exam that they took at a young age in part defines who they are. Children are simmered in this all-encompassing, high-stakes personal pressure for years and years.

We saw earlier that unhappiness with schoolwork is one of the key factors accounting for children's deteriorating mental health.[33] We can understand this more through some recent research in the USA looking at 'high-achieving schools'. This showed four major risk factors for mental illness in adolescence.[lxxxix] The first three – poverty, trauma and discrimination – are not a surprise; they show what we have always known about mental illness: that deprivation takes

---

33 Interestingly, the second area that shows up in their annual survey is an unhappiness with appearance, which is likely related to the impact that viewing 'perfect' bodies on social media has on body dissatisfaction. As I say, this mental-health crisis is not about one thing; it is about different types of pressure acting in combination.

its toll. But the fourth was new information: it showed that attending a high-achieving school is also a risk factor. The privileged kids, with all the opportunities, are showing up with high levels of anxiety and depression – six or seven times the national norm.

Why are these privileged kids suffering at these schools? It doesn't seem to be as simple as high-achieving schools exerting massive pressure on their pupils who then become mentally unwell; or perhaps it doesn't seem to be *just* that. The researchers argue that the different systems act together to create a damaging environment: that these schools attract the 'squeezed middle' parents who are drawn to them as they are ambitious for their kids in the context of increased global competition. The schools, keen to meet parental ambitions, stretch each child to seek distinction and reach their highest potential. The students, likely a genetically bright bunch, compare themselves to their high-achieving peers, and compete for positions in top sets and best colleges, which acts to undermine the friendships and support that would normally ameliorate a high-pressure environment. In combination, these factors create a competitive survival-of-the-fittest mentality in the children, which damages their mental health. As I said, this research was conducted in America, but I don't think it's too much of a leap from there to a UK context, or other countries of the world. Certainly, in my clinical practice, I see a lot of kids like those in the US, who, as the researchers put it, 'are experiencing unrelenting pressure to accomplish ever more and distinguish themselves as among the best'.[xc]

I am reminded of Ken Robinson's words in his 2016 TED Talk:[34]

---

[34] Ken Robinson was a professor of education, and his TED Talk on whether schools kill creativity is one of the most watched of all time.

Academic ability . . . has really come to dominate our view of intelligence, because the universities designed the system in their image. If you think of it, the whole system of public education around the world is a protracted process of university entrance. And the consequence is that many highly talented, brilliant, creative people think they're not, because the thing they were good at at school wasn't valued or was actually stigmatised.

As Ken Robinson captures, much of the pressure at school is to achieve the grades for a place at a 'good' university, and I am struck in my clinics by how many young people are working relentlessly, without joy, to chase this. The hyperbole about top universities, largely coming from themselves, maintains a system of exclusivity that damages many.[35] It seems like a squid game of academic achievement to see who can put in the most hours of studying in a day. The hard-work-conquers-all and other messages of personal responsibility make it an exercise in endurance for so many. I fear that the situation has got worse, not better, since Ken Robinson gave his talk: the hours put in for top achievement are no longer a rehearsal for an academic life; they are, instead, becoming a test of whether you are suited to doing all-nighters in a city law firm or corporate finance, rather than a test of innate ability, intellectual curiosity or interest. Teachers become experts at teaching to the test to obtain the best possible outcomes for their pupils – unlocking the exam-passing code, but at what cost?

---

35 The Russell Group is a self-appointed, self-regulated group and does not involve any external monitoring of best. Please see my book *You Don't Understand Me* for further thoughts on this point.

THE PERFECT STORM – THE ADOLESCENT YEARS

I was interested to see Sam Carling, one of our new 2024 young MPs, reflecting on his time at Cambridge University: 'The university had a huge problem with mental health. If you put a lot of high achievers in one place, you know what's going to happen.'[xci] Well, Sam, *you* might know that, but I don't think it's widely understood, given the numbers who apply. It also damages many of the Oxbridge rejects, of whom there are over 30,000 a year, previously feted as the top of their schools, singled out for awards and prizes, some of whom have been chasing this dream for years. When I see them, they hold a sense of not being good enough, which is very hard to shift, and which, I suspect for many, is quite untrue: they were perhaps just unlucky. My observation is that this mass-competition education system isn't good for anyone. The competitive attitude becomes embedded, so young people feel they should strive to the limits of their academic ability and for high status, rather than what they want to or can comfortably do.

Parents can get sucked into being too invested in this process, with their child's outcome or progress at the front of their minds, and seeing their primary role as to support that. Kids have daily tutoring, or live-in tutors, and yet the parents say they are not 'pushy' – they just want to support their child to do their best. 'Best' here seems to mean the very peak of their academic achievement, even though this requires a 24/7 commitment, and is not necessarily the child's natural path or a level they can sustain in the longer term independently. Parents doing this amplify the pressure from school or university, and, as I discussed in Chapter 3.2, that undermines the manifesto for mental health. The US research referred to earlier backs this up. They found 'parents seeking perfection' through 'criticism and expectations' was a key factor for differentiating which kids who attended high-achieving schools ended up suffering with mental illness.[xcii] Even if kids avoid mental ill health they can end up performing at a level they can't maintain comfortably: they continue to need parental or tutor support when they are at university, or even when they start work.

I hope we are beginning to see a backlash against this achievement-above-all mindset. Perhaps cognisant that many are achieving beyond their natural ability through extreme means, firms are moving to blind recruitment, where they don't have access to information such as which school or university applicants attended. I read with optimism that Wall Street firms are beginning to recruit beyond the traditional Ivy League colleges: great people don't always get the top grades at eighteen.[36]

THE INTERNET AND SOCIAL MEDIA

So where are we? We know that adolescents tend to compare and contrast themselves in the search for an identity. We also know that the education system has become more competitive, test-orientated, outcome-focused, with more subdivisions of excellence. And that this reflects societal attitudes about achievement, busyness and outcome. Then, into this heady mix, in tween and teenage years, we drop the bomb that is social media.

Now, don't get me wrong, social media can be a good and positive place, allowing groups of friends to connect and share warmth and humour. It also can create a sense of belonging, particularly for marginalised groups to find each other and offer support. It can be a creative place, where funny memes

---

36 It is fair to say that I am a person with a vested interest in that point of view.

or TikTok dance crazes pass around the world in hours. There is stuff to like about social media, and I've written about this before.[xciii]

But sadly, social media is not just about connecting friends – it is also about comparison. Indeed, it is a perfectly designed platform for searching out improved versions of yourself to negatively compare yourself to. Smartphones – such a visual and quick medium – make the process of comparison supercharged. No longer do you just have to compare yourself to your class, school year or local community, as we did a generation ago – there are now infinite examples of otherness, betterness, always available, creating a worldwide competition and heightening the feeling of not being good enough.

Social media can naturally amplify the most difficult bits of being a tween or teenager: we see this in the social media starter drug, WhatsApp. Whilst parents see it as a relatively harmless communication tool, allowing groups of friends to connect, it can actually be a formal platform that amplifies the problems of the on-off friend and the triangulation of friendships that we discussed previously. For example, girls A, B and C have a WhatsApp group; A also has one with B (where they talk about C) and one with C (where they talk about B). B and C have one, in theory, but rarely use it in practice, as they are both competing for the good attention of A.

As adolescents progress through the social media chain, through Snapchat, Instagram, TikTok, these sorts of friendship issues are ingrained into the structure of these platforms: they are built on inclusion and exclusion, likes or their absence, messages opened or not, ghosting. This means real-life tensions can be heightened by the core design of the platforms. There is no respite from them either – playground fights gain traction online overnight, rather than dissipating as they did back in the day when there was only a landline to communicate, and *nobody* called after 9pm. Social media is peer pressure on speed.

Social media can also intensify the normal adolescent-appearance awareness. Adolescents nowadays, particularly girls, are seeing thousands more images of how they 'should' look. This can push the normal self-consciousness a teenage girl has about her appearance through the stratosphere. It largely promotes an unachievable level of 'beauty', especially through the use of filters and editing, but also because for the stars of social media beauty, fitness and slimness are their full-time job. They encourage girls into beauty and fitness regimes that are unachievable within normal lives or budgets. The research on the impact of this is unequivocal. Viewing so-called perfect bodies online or in other media impacts negatively on body satisfaction, which, in turn, can contribute to anxiety and eating disorders.[xciv] Normal adolescent self-consciousness can be pushed into self-obsession and dissatisfaction.

For boys, the patterns can be a bit different. We saw that they game more, and we have seen this can be linked to aggression. We also know that most teenagers have viewed violent porn by the age of eighteen years old, and that the frequency of this is linked with violent sexual acts.[xcv] Boys who don't feel good enough can be attracted to the money and status of misogynists like Andrew Tate, adopting a persona of bluster and superiority to hide a fear of inferiority – a fear of being undesirable or not enough.[xcvi]

The thing is, when we raise children to think in comparative terms, in a do-better-and-get-more culture, in adolescence, we no longer control what they compare to or want to do better and get more of. As they search for identity and become self-conscious about their bodies, they may search for more and better of the 'wrong' things: extreme eating, beauty or fitness regimes, more extreme porn, more violence, more gratuitous displays of wealth or success . . .

These are just some examples of how the internet and social media can be catalysts for the normal trials and tribulations of adolescence, increasing image dissatisfaction, encouraging aggression, warping an interest in sex. I touch on just a few issues here, because the myriad of others have been well covered elsewhere. But, unlike some commenters, I do not see social media as the whole problem. Indeed, I think screens have become the scapegoat that enables us to avoid looking at the more painful aspects of our own parenting and the society we have created. It is uncomfortable for us to look at what we might have done in this last generation to feed this mental-health crisis: simpler to wholeheartedly blame the phone.

PERFECT PARENTING STANDARDS

What is emerging here, in part, is a story of striving for high or perfect standards on many different levels, in schools and on social media, which amplifies the normal adolescent process of seeking an identity through comparison. And one of the ways it is amplified is when parents hold perfectionistic standards themselves.

Perfectionism, you will remember, is the constant striving for higher standards whilst judging yourself (or others) harshly. In this book, we've so far considered how it can impact your parenting in the baby years, in feeding your child or in your approach to school; but it is not just about these areas; relentlessly high, judgy standards can occur in many different scenarios.

Many people, it seems, are proud to be perfectionists. They humble boast about it: 'I am a perfectionist', they say; they believe that their perfectionism has steered them on to higher standards, more wealth and success, a better body. They seem to overestimate the influence of their hard work and efforts in this, and underestimate the role of things like luck, innate ability, being born in the right place and right time.[xcvii] They also don't dwell on the negative effects of perfectionism; they like only to see the positives. They are like someone who has smoked their whole life but doesn't believe the link with lung cancer because they haven't got it; and then, if they do get it, they blame it on genetics or something else. They believe in the motivational benefits of perfectionism – that they 'deserve' their success because they worked so hard for it. Perfectionism really does have great PR.

I want to make a distinction, though. If a grown adult is perfectionistic, either by nature or nurture, and thinks it is of benefit and doesn't try to change it, that's on them. If they are a parent, that is different. Because whether or not they are damaging themselves is one thing; but they may be imposing those attitudes on their children. Back to lung cancer again. If you as an adult want to smoke, that's on you. If you impose passive smoking on your children; that's a different thing; you are endangering them.

Children can inherit a parent's perfectionism through both genetics and social-learning.[xcviii, xcix] Just as kids whose parents smoke are three times more likely to smoke themselves, children of perfectionists can absorb the self-controlled, striving mentality of busyness, deprivation and seeking the best through this being the norm in their childhood. Now, of course, there is little to do about the genetic predispositions we pass on, but parents can and should take responsibility for perfectionism expression in front of their children.

Parental perfectionism can impact on children and adolescents to worsen mental health, as it undermines the framework elements.[c] We have seen this throughout the book. How it can mess with the baby–parent attachment, by creating an asynchronicity between them, and that can be damaging, as the attachment relationship is the blueprint for all future relationships. We've seen how expecting behavioural control with younger children can make us over-controlling or critical (in framework terms, too firm), and for adolescents and young adults criticism and control are the major pathways for parental perfectionism to translate into adolescent distress.[ci] We've seen how with food and eating, parents might give a constant stream of instructions and standards that live in a child's head and which disconnect them from their own intuition and nutritional needs. And we've seen all through the book how the anxiety perfectionism causes parents is contagious for their children, increasing the likelihood that they too will be anxious. Finally, in this chapter, we've seen how parents can amplify high academic striving in a system of pressure with school and peers to increase the likelihood of mental illness.[cii]

Here, I want to make another distinction, and that is between two types of perfectionism. The first is *self-orientated perfectionism*: a perfection you direct towards yourself. That shows a mixed picture in the research – whilst there may be some positive motivational benefits, there are a whole heap of negative ones, too, including burnout and a link to early death.[ciii] When parents impress perfect standards on their children, that is the more toxic *socially prescribed perfectionism* that we touched on earlier in Chapter 3.1, 'The Busyness Business'. Here, the baby/child/adolescent isn't coming to perfectionism through their own personality, life experience and autonomy – they are having it imposed upon them by their parents, and by the current social environment. So self-orientated perfectionism has some major disadvantages, but nothing like those of having perfectionism thrust upon you by your parents, as well as the rest of society, from the time you are a tiny baby.

A perfect parent risks implanting the observer's voice in children's heads by giving them standards to meet and constant feedback on their attempts to do so. Their young people can end up hooked on the opinions of others, and often not know their own. This is what I hear is in so many of the minds of the young people I see in therapy – what they ruminate and introspect on are the actual or perceived opinions of others to the point that their self-esteem exists entirely outside of themselves. They don't think, 'I did this well. I like this – I am proud of it.' Rather, they think, 'But what do other people want of me and think of this?' Their very own version of how-do-I-want-to-be-seen haunts their lives. And when they reach adolescence, wired as they are to look away from you, their parent, they will use this mindset in their interactions with others who (unlike you) might not have their best interests at heart. People on Tik-Tok, for example, or a controlling partner, a toxic friend, a bullying boss. You may have unwittingly trained them to look for that person's good opinion, too. This type of socially prescribed perfectionism – yearning for the good opinion of others – contributes to anxiety, depression, self-harm, obsessive-compulsive disorder, suicidal ideation and burnout.

And, sadly, I don't think this is a problem for just the most extreme perfect parents I have caricatured in this book. I think this is a zeitgeist problem, where ideas about constant self-improvement have embedded themselves in us all. There has been a ratcheting up of our involvement in our children's lives, often with an ambitious agenda. Most of the parents I see in clinic are absolutely lovely. They are often the sort of people who give me faith in humanity and inspire me to be a 'better' person myself. They might have stacks of patience, or an incredible drive to stay positive, or are dripping with kindness. They have kept the rules of life; they have celebrated and encouraged their child's every success, their appearance, their talent. They have been engaged, involved in every aspect of their child's life, and have praised, and guided, and channelled and opined. They've just wanted the best for their children: they've wanted them to achieve where they themselves haven't. They've taken their children's education seriously, hired tutors, helped with homework. They've wanted to guide and nurture, perhaps in areas where they themselves were left to figure everything out on their own. They've wanted to manage their children's behaviour kindly, where perhaps they were overlooked, under-supported or, worse, treated harshly as kids. They've made themselves crucial to their adolescent's forward trajectory and are always on the other end of the ubiquitous phone for cheerleading or problem-solving.

They've done all this, unaware that in the context of a fast-paced, better-and-more society, the internet and social media and an outcome-based education system, they were unwittingly adding to the storm of opinion and approval around their child – a storm that seems to be battering many young people to bits. They were adding fuel to the fire of expectation that surrounds our children and contributes to a striving, best-seeking attitude that undermines their mental health.[civ] It is in this way, I believe, that our society has shifted along a mental-health continuum towards poorer mental health.

THE GOOD-ENOUGH PARENT IN ADOLESCENCE
And so, in light of all this pressure trickling down through society, including from the education system and social media, and an adolescent primed to self-compare, I am arguing that you

should choose to be a good-enough parent, not an extreme one. Not one obsessing about the nutritional quality of all their food or getting them into the very best school; nor micro-managing their work or taking every spelling test super seriously. This is why you need to not be setting out schedules of activities, nor grading all their behaviour through sticker charts. Not spending twenty-four hours with them with skin-on-skin contact, expecting the perfect attachment bond. This is why you are not expecting 100 per cent compliance in their behaviour, or that their rooms are meticulous. You need to be teaching them good-enough by example. Because everything else around them is giving them another false and often unhelpful message of self-improvement, and if you add to this, rather than mitigate it, I believe you could be putting the setting conditions together for your child to suffer mentally.

The good-enough parents are, on the surface, less 'good'. They may be slightly less involved in their children's lives and have a more hands-off style, which promotes independence and autonomy. Hands off, but not neglectful, of course. This is the messy middle, not down the other end of the continuum, near abuse. They make plenty of time to be together, for fun, for empathy and for curiosity. They are also not afraid to get involved where necessary, to set boundaries and be firm, and are prepared to be unpopular in the short term. But they use these skills sparingly and wisely. They do, of course, care deeply about their children (most parents do), but they believe that children find their own way, and that imposing stuff on them is largely counterproductive. So they give their opinion a little less often, holding back a bit on praise or sanction: they don't want to fill their adolescent with their views, but want them to have space to find their own. They are wise enough to know that the only motivation that works is self-motivation:

you can't push kids into self-orientated perfectionism, with its potential motivational benefits; you can only drive them into socially prescribed perfectionism, which is just toxic. You can't push kids into success either, and a good-enough parent doesn't get over-invested in their children's success or failure but will always be there to support them get over the important hurdles. To return to Gary Lineker's sideline analogy (see p. 126): the good-enough parent is watching the game with benign interest, looking for the joy and fun, but not over-invested in how their child plays or whether they win or not. They are sensitive to how their child is feeling about the game afterwards, rather than offering coaching tips. They will, of course, spend a couple of hours in goal if their kid wants to practise, but they won't suggest that they need to, or be nagging them to do so. They will also be mindful about when it's time to stop practising – when enough is enough.

You see, as a parent, you do not control the societal message, education policy, the friends they meet. You should try, but are unlikely to be wholly successful, to control the content they get from the internet. You don't control their outcome, their personality or their path. But you do control one important thing: you control your own attitude, and through this, you can demonstrate and live an approach of good enough, with a messier house, a less-good craft project and a less illustrious career, but more balance, joy and stronger relationships. You can let go of trying to control their path, but instead, enjoy walking alongside them, altering your route to accompany them on theirs when they need you to. You can support them to achieve but believe that if you give them a secure base, they will find their own best way. You can *trust them* to find their own way. You can remember that appearance is secondary to substance. That excellence is less important than connection. You can teach them all about the fun of imperfection by example. In this way, you will optimise manifesto aims: helping them to feel good enough; having a capacity for happiness and low anxiety; they will have had the best setting conditions for independence, and you will not have damaged your relationship with them by imposing your standards on them.

I'm going to think about the sixth manifesto aim – emotional competence – for just a bit longer, though. You see, good-enough parenting might appear a bit lazy, a bit hands-off, a bit low effort, even a bit selfish, but actually the opposite is true. I am going to say being good enough is always a bit tricky, much harder than the fake clarity of perfection, extremity and certainty. At the start of the book, I gave you the analogy that good-enough parenting is like standing at the centre of a see-saw in a state of constant flux to find balance, as opposed to sitting at either end, where your position is held firm. This is never more true than in your child's adolescent years. In part, they find their identity by questioning yours, and your parenting, and that means you have to self-reflect and adjust as necessary.

It can, at times, be a struggle when you feel you are second guessing yourself: am I giving enough support to scaffold them, but not taking over? Am I encouraging a good learning environment without stressing on their outcome? Am I being firm enough that they are safe, without either being mean or negating their independence? Good enough is subtle and nuanced, and that doesn't make it an easy choice. It means staying engaged and alert in a different way: monitoring and adjusting to adapt to your child's path and the relationship space between you, rather than forcing them on to your predetermined path. It's like the reciprocity and synchronicity we saw in goo-goo-gah-gah parenting in a different form – responding to your adolescent as an individual, whilst still providing warmth and boundaries. Hopefully, you and your co-parent can help each other find the balance; or, if not, find a supportive, good-enough friend to discuss it all with.

So it is in this parental struggle, where you acknowledge the disparities, the contradictions and the individuality of your adolescent, and allow them to push back a bit against you, that I think their emotional competence is built. You are not pretending it is easy or that you have all the answers; you are bearing uncertainty, which, as we know, is the key to a low-anxiety life. But you are staying steady, like the ballast in the storm of an increasingly extreme and fractured world, which will help them learn to cope with that. You are showing up honestly, vulnerably in your relationship with them, not always right or certain, and in that way, you teach by example the emotional competence they are going to need.

Because as you get to late adolescence, you will find that your relationship with them is really the only important tool you have left to support and guide them. I will explore how that works in the chapter after next. First, let's go for one last time to 'firm and kind' and think about how they play out with different types of adolescents, and why firm particularly is on diminishing returns over these crucial years.

4.2
Holding On and Letting Go

In the last chapter, we looked at how being a good-enough parent helps a child to be free to develop their own identity, separate from the swirling storm of opinion that surrounds them. This chapter is dominated by another key task of adolescent development, that of separation, and this links directly to the manifesto aim of independence. Your role as a parent is to raise a child who is competent – emotionally, financially and practically – and able to leave you. This separation is a bit like a pendulum swing – they swing further away from you in teenage years and swing part-way back to establish the right distance for adulthood. That can make the teenage years a time of storm and stress – both theirs and yours – but this pushing off by them is part of the process of establishing a healthy adult-to-adult relationship in the future.

During the secondary-school years, children's independence from their parents generally grows naturally. They will likely develop a separate world you know nothing about, and the evolutionary drive is away from you. They tend to stop wanting to spend as much time with you: they stop wanting you to read them a story at night, they eschew 'family movie night' to go out with their friends, and other nights they disappear into their bedroom on their phone or computer. It's the beginning of their attachments to new friends and interests.

Whilst the technology is new, the distancing is completely natural. There will have been moments of separation before, when they toddled off from you at a playgroup or their first day at school or even the first time you left them at someone else's house for a party or playdate, but in the adolescent years, the pace of this speeds up. They spend more time away from you, more often. It is important to remember as a parent that this separating from you is a crucial part of their development: making strong bonds with their peers is the first step of a process that continues through finding a mate (or mates), getting a job, leaving home. As parents, we can sometimes scoff at the importance friends take on, but, in a million of these bonds up and down the country, and increasingly, through social media, around the world, they are forging their generation: the commonalities of experience and language that act as a springboard for the world to progress.

Before secondary school, it is as though they are on a long bit of elastic, and every day they ping back to you. In secondary school, that elastic stretches beyond rapid recoil and is at risk of breaking. You want a strong thread there through adult life, but never again will you have the closeness of a young child. By the end of secondary school, they are legal adults, if not emotionally and financially independent ones.

How do you feel about that?

If you are reading this with a younger child, you may feel pre-emptively sad at the thought that you will one day lose the closeness of your family nest. Some of you may react with a heavy heart or dread at the thought that they will grow – or have grown – apart from you. You may fear the emptiness of loss that their growing up will leave. For some of you there may be a sense of sadness that a stage of your life that you loved is over – no more finger painting, long days at the park or playing doll's house for hours. For others, perhaps those of you already deep in the teenage years, that may be met with a sense of joy or relief, of freedom, of getting your life back. Many of you probably feel contradictory emotions about this separation.

It is important to look at your own feelings about this as these will undoubtedly play out in your parenting. As I said in the identity chapter (1.4), I don't buy any assumption that we, as parents, respond to our children in a wholly rational way, devoid of our own psychological make-up, to maximise a successful outcome. It is the myth of the perfect parent and the infantilised child, positioning parents as all knowing, totally reasonable, emotionally calm and always right. It's not what I see in clinic, and it's not what I see in myself. Most of the parents I meet of troubled adolescents are perfectly lovely, and usually utterly committed to their children, but their emotional history and current needs are playing out in the theatre of family life. That isn't to say they are to blame or at fault in their child's difficulties – as we've seen, this is not a simple-factor storm – but, as I've previously discussed, parental psychology and identity is one factor in their child's experience.

And as the crucial task of adolescence is separation and individuation from parents, and for a parent that involves letting go of them, that can be really hard on you both emotionally and practically. At ten or eleven years old, as you prepare your child for secondary school, you will likely still be super involved, arranging playdates with other local kids going to the same school, going uniform or outfit shopping or testing out the bus route to the new school. But the direction of their travel is not limited just to the bus route; emotionally, it will be away from you to independence, and part of your job is to keep your eye on that horizon.

After they start at big school, probably relatively quickly, you will not know who they are playing and hanging out with. Next, will be the way they look or how they dress. Issues of safety will likely rear their heads in the later teens, with them rebelling about how late they stay out or how they get home, or drugs and alcohol. Emotionally, letting go of all those areas of responsibility is a loss for you: a loss of a role and a loss of an identity. The cost of their freedom to explore their identity is the space you need to give to them, and that may mean that you feel less close to them. But even if your kid takes a less traditional 'teenage' path, and isn't a party animal, it is important that they have areas of separation, whether that's about their political views or religious beliefs or what they study. It's sometimes the quiet ones who can't rebel that you need to worry about, as the need to separate is like a boiling pot with the lid on, and the fire still burning. It can bubble over and come out in some form or other – repressive ways like OCD or anorexia.

Practically, this is not an easy time either. Behavioural theory, and the parenting gurus who preach that ethos, would have consistency as the be all and end all of behaviour management. But this becomes nonsensical in the face of child development, and the pace of that accelerates in the teenage years. How is consistency possible when they, and their social world, are changing all the time? For example, you might set a rule that you don't want them staying out till 11pm at age fourteen. But then another parent asks them on a special theatre trip, and you say yes. Then the next week, it is a cinema trip, which you don't think is quite as justifiable, but you agree, as it is almost the same as a theatre trip. But really how different is that to them watching a movie at that friend's house? And then what if they are in that parent's home, but there are other teenagers there? But then, next time, it is a different parent's home, one of the down-with-the-kids-no-boundaries kind of parents. Should you be discriminating between parents, really? It is often a war of attrition; kids wear us down by these types of gradations. The complexity and nuance are endless and, of course, we have to adjust to their age and changing circumstances. We can't be consistent because time is a dimension that changes everything.

So the terrain of separation and individuation has two axes: the parents' and the adolescents'. The first axis is how well parents facilitate their child's autonomy: at the extremes, do they hold on too tight or let go too easily? Firm and kind are intrinsically caught up in this. The second axis is the child's drive to autonomy and independence, and that runs from adolescents who rebel at one end to those who fear separation at the other.

What can possibly go wrong?

WHAT HAPPENS WHEN YOU HOLD ON TOO TIGHT ...

The problems I see in my clinics in relation to adolescent separation and individuation fall, as they often do, at opposite ends of a continuum.

Frequently, I see that the extremity in parenting that I've been tracing throughout this book, where a parent is focused on achieving the best outcome for their child, keeps the child infantilised or pushes them into rebellion. For parents like this, their adolescent's life is always a work in progress, needing their involvement and input. There is often an over-interest in their child's academic progress; adolescents and young adults never reach a finish line – they are always on to the next target, and some, possibly many, parents over-invest in this. Parents like this are struggling to let go of being firm – and that can be because of their own emotions rather than the child's.

In early adolescence, that might look like too many rules, not adjusting to their child's new friends or interests, wanting their child to continue with their old activities. In older adolescence, I see late teens or young adults being 'parented' too much; parents stepping too frequently or too quickly into their child's life: the focus is often on their outcome, and there is an uber amount of academic pressure, their timetables and routines are protected and they do not take on the rites of passage of doing chores or their own laundry, cooking simple meals or earning their own money. These are seen as less important than the project of self-improvement. Instead, children graduate from adult-led play activities, such as their swim team or tennis camp, to the pretend 'work' of work experience or volunteering. In middle-class life, this has become the norm in society and so, as parents, we tend to go along with it, ruefully raising an eyebrow and lamenting on the benefits we got in our own teenage years from the paper round we did or the café we waited in, whilst mining our contacts for a suitable work-experience week.

The parent who is holding on too tight is preventing adolescents developing the key skills they need to be an adult. They are struggling to allow their child the space to find their own autonomy and competence. Autonomy is a sense of freedom to make their own decisions, and indeed make their own mistakes, which has been linked to so many mental- and physical-health benefits. Autonomy is key to adolescents feeling respected – and the irony, of course, is that when adolescents feel respected, they actually comply better.[cv] In the research literature, autonomy is associated with all the positive stuff: resilience, coping in the face of stress and even longevity itself.[cvi]

Sometimes this has been posited in parental advice as allowing children opportunities to fail. And indeed, being able to fail with grace and move forwards is an important life skill.

Roger Federer has spoken about how he lost 46 per cent of the points he played – lots of failing goes into winning. But I hate creating fake opportunities to fail for young people or bigging up failure on the way to success; and young people don't fall for that bullshit anyway. I think this is really about two things: one I touched on earlier is giving them opportunities not to compete, but the second is what I was discussing in the perfect-storm chapter: the opportunity to make their own choices without opinion or judgment. To find their own intrinsic motivation from within, and not feel coerced into something by the direct pressure of being told to do it or the indirect pressure of fearing parental disappointment or disapproval.

Parents who think they are responsible for their adolescents' outcome are likely to be highly anxious: it is anxiety provoking thinking you are responsible for the outcome of a whole separate adult. If you are thinking about your adolescent all the time, wanting them to achieve, worrying about their UCAS personal statement or what time they are home at night, you are going to be pretty anxious. And when humans are anxious, they seek control. But this runs contrary to your adolescent's natural drive to separate and individuate. This disparity is a problem because adolescents then have to rebel too hard or suppress the urge to separate to cope with their parent's anxiety, and we will see how that plays out later in the chapter. Parents – and I hate to be disloyal to my gender, but in my experience it is mainly mums – sometimes use that anxiety to justify their behavioural control, saying things like, 'I need them in before I go to sleep', to defend a curfew. No – they don't *need* that, they *want* it. Your anxiety should not be your adolescent's problem. The love you need to practise now is the love of letting go.

The real answer should be letting go of your adolescent–adult, bearing in mind that they are separating from you and will soon be leaving, that they are a whole person with their own thoughts, beliefs and values – someone over whom you now have little control. That is uncomfortable – painful, even – but it also is necessary for your child's independent life and your relationship with them.

. . . OR NOT TIGHT ENOUGH?

At the other end of the continuum are those parents who give up on any illusion of boundaries as soon as their child can get a bus to school on their own. In later years, they often befriend their child, smoking a joint at the kitchen table with their friends, letting a succession of boy-/girlfriends sleep over. This chapter is about letting go and holding on, and boundaries are crucially important in teenage years. If I judged the state of the nation from my clinical work, holding too tight is more frequently a problem currently in society, but having no boundaries is probably worse for any individual child than having too many. Whilst some boundary-less kids end up super sensible, like Saffy in *Absolutely Fabulous*, many seem to be taking ket and sleeping around at thirteen. It can feel for an adolescent that their parents just don't care when they aren't prepared to set the boundaries.

Because loving a kid in adolescence is about them finding their way and you both adapting to that, but also holding on to some of the containment discussed in Chapter 3.4 on internet and screens. Containment, as you may remember, helps kids feel safe and secure. It gives them boundaries on their behaviour, which means that they are hopefully not going to fuck up too badly, doing anything irretrievably awful or permanent. But when you do put boundaries in place, you are setting yourself up, as the parent of an adolescent, as a dartboard – and giving them the darts. Parenting with boundaries may mean being ridiculed, scorned and mocked for being out of touch, for not being as cool as the other parents. But it is also to keep loving when you are being shouted at, told that they hate you and are slamming the door. Parents who don't set boundaries try to avoid this – they want things to be nice and easy. Again, their emotions may be playing out in their parenting. Sometimes they are not securely attached themselves – and so they fear the conflict or rejection that happens when you set boundaries.

I'm not saying this is simple or easy, and indeed, as we will go on to see, some children are more and others less compliant, but I am saying some boundaries are important. One week, in clinic, I saw two families with similar problems in that their daughters had eating disorders and didn't want to eat dinner. One was thirteen and the other was nineteen. The family of the thirteen-year-old said, 'How can we make her eat?' and so their daughter skipped off without food to hang out with her friends in the park. The other daughter told me, 'My parents made me have it.' I asked them how they did this, and they said they told her she had to. They would have taken the car keys away if she had tried to go out without eating, but they didn't have to say that – she complied. The two different attitudes came from the parents (a reluctance to set boundaries vs an expectation of compliance), but also from the children. Some are lower and others higher on accepting their parents' legitimacy to parent; and indeed, they are lower or higher on their inclination to obey. Let's have a think about that.

KIDS WHO PUSH AT THE BOUNDARIES
As a parent, I remember one day in late summer with my three in my car, pulling over in tears on the drive to a park. I said (wailed?) to one of them, 'You haven't done one thing first time I've told you this whole school holiday'. It was true.

My other two sometimes ignore me, busy in their own world or playing for time over something they don't want to do. Maybe I get compliance half of the time on the first time of asking. My third child, though, is in a different category: you've met him before in the toddler tantrums and internet and screens chapters. He pulls away from any authority or semblance of compliance at all. With a child like this, everything feels like a fight. They fundamentally do not recognise the parents' legitimacy to parent, and so lack any inclination to obey. This is a type of child that's seared on my soul. Kids like this just don't accept the implicit social contract that adults are in charge. And they are hard to parent. If you have one, you may think they are the hardest of all, but I guess I would argue that with this kind of kid you are getting what is on the tin. The dilemma, the struggle, the conflict – it is all in the open; indeed, by adolescence, they are shouting it in your face, telling you it is your fault; and why don't you just fuck off anyway. They argue with you all the time: you say black, they say white; you say up, they say down.

Why? Well, they don't agree with the social hierarchy, but they also seem to push against whatever it is saying to figure out their own identity. The sense I get of their unconscious self is that it is an affront to their identity that you would even say whatever you say; that you are offending them by inflicting your opinion on them; that for their own sense of integrity they now have to do the opposite. Note, I say unconscious self: half the time they will seemingly argue without even knowing why they are doing so. They didn't even know they cared until you said the opposite.

The risk in your parenting is twofold: a rebellious child with a parent who doesn't hold on tight enough can be a recipe for an adolescent spiralling into some extreme behaviours as there is nothing stopping them. But at the other end of the continuum, a parent who holds on too tight, well, the risks are there that you allow their intransigence to damage the relationship between you, which again can lead to rebellion: remember the toddler-tantrum literature, where time out was followed with a slap or the child being put in the closet with the entrance barred? It is the same spiralling up with an adolescent: if you parent them relying on firm, you end up going head to head, threatening to take their phone away, for an hour, for a day, then a week, then a month, then a year, because they are telling you that they don't care anyway, and are challenging you to do it. As it spirals, you can find yourself threatening to smash the bloody thing with a hammer because, say, at the start of all this, they didn't empty the dishwasher. Going head to head with them in an argument is like putting them in a metaphorical closet and barring the entrance: they can't get out, they can't back down and they hate being trapped. Don't get me wrong. They care deeply about your good opinion of them, but they want your good opinion to be about the core of them, and not about their compliance with your silly rules. They will only back down if you break their spirit or you frighten them.

And do we want to do this? No, we do not. We may find ourselves doing it because they are so exasperating, but we should try not to. As parents, we can often feel undervalued by society, as well as our nearest and dearest, but don't even try to get your sense of worth, your sense of being listened to, from arguing with your child or adolescent if they are like this. You are just going to feel worse. Why go head to head with anyone if they are never going to back down? You need to be smarter than that. Outwit, outlast, outplay.

It may help you to keep in mind that their obstinacy is fundamentally a good thing: it is the other side of them being determined, having grit and banging their own drum. These are exasperating qualities to parent, but excellent ones to have in adulthood. Your kid is driven by their own opinion, rather than that of others. This is the autonomy we were talking of earlier; their behaviour being driven by their own interests, goals and values, and less so by external pressure. It is an internal locus of control: they see themselves and not you as being responsible for their life. But they can't have autonomy and a good relationship with you if they sense or you express your disapproval of their decisions and choices. Your disapproval plays on their mind and warps either their autonomy or your relationship, so use it wisely. We will see in the next chapter how it's important not to use up your disapproval on the small stuff (tidying rooms) or the stuff that is frankly none of your business (what subjects they choose to study).

Whilst you are parenting them, what with the arguing back and the defiance in the face of your boundaries, you may fear that they are going to turn into a dictator or a psychopath. You may feel you need to break their spirit, and find yourself arguing yourself into a corner, where neither of you can back down. But actually, this is the exact behaviour that will make them more of a dictator, as it will stoke their simmering rage at the unfairness of it all. What you need to do is try not to squash it out of them. Give them a way out, hug them tight and love them really hard, even though they will never agree with you. *Show* them how to back down, how to de-escalate, how to get out of a situation with their pride intact. You don't have to agree, but you can be calmish, firmish, and as kind as you can be in the face of their rudeness and disobedience. Humour sometimes helps.

They will push every boundary. This is how it plays out. You say 10pm; they come in at 10.30, with you going through half an hour of radio silence. You feel like shouting and grounding them for a month. Don't. If you do, they won't keep to it – they will climb out of their window, and then you will get into punishment-escalation mode. Instead, take a deep breath and lead with 'Did you have a nice evening?' and genuinely listen to their answer. You are leading with 'relationship' and 'kind'. Then, as you are leaving the room to go to bed, say, 'Next time please come in nearer ten'. There then will be a list of seven reasons why they were late – none of them will be their fault – and an eighth: why it's a stupid rule anyway. Listen, neutral faced, don't get sucked into arguing, repeat the rule and get out: 'Yes, it does sound frustrating that someone else lost your bus pass/that Sophie had a drama you needed to sort/that your phone was on silent, but none the less, I do expect you home at ten. Goodnight, darling, I'm off to bed. Turn off the lights on your way up. Love you!'

My guess is that the lights will be on in the morning, and that they will continue to come home at 10.30, but they are unlikely to come home at 1am because you are maintaining your relationship with them, and they love and care about you, and really don't want to piss you off because they do value their bond with you. If you don't do this, and if you regularly shout and punish them, then you will lose the little control you do have through goodwill – through your relationship. Kids comply more when they feel valued and respected. If you lose the relationship in their head – if they think you don't love them anyway – why bother to comply at all?

These are adolescents. You need to parent by example, not by winning the argument. By my children's adolescence, I had started to learn this lesson. I'd begun to (sometimes) walk out of the room when I was beginning to lose it – not stomp out, but just go somewhere else when something wasn't worth getting cross about. It was a little win in my head the other day as I heard my kids say to each other when I'd left the room because it was all too annoying, 'Yeah, but I think it's pissing Mum off.' I'd taught them to reflect on the opinions and feelings of others, not through arguing my point to the nth degree or wielding my power and control, but through quiet self-restraint. I try to divert the argument till it can be a discussion and not a row. I accept that with semi-adults (who are allowed to have jobs, sex, leave school, drive) I'm not going to get it all my own way. I'm teaching them the negotiation and empathy of adult relationships, rather than the idea that I am an all-knowing, always-right control freak.[37] I maintain my right to have the final say on stuff about the house and family as a whole, but not so much about their lives.

The issue is keeping hold of them enough that they don't mess up and maintaining your relationship whilst you do. You will be biting your lip. Personally, I am still a work in progress on this. *sigh*

THE GOOD GIRL – WHAT HAPPENS WHEN THEY ARE TOO POLITE TO REJECT YOU?

I said above that the boundary-pusher was a hard kid to parent, but at least you know what you are getting with them. The kid who won't rebel and is determined to be 'good', whilst secretly self-harming, is a more unknown quantity and arguably harder to parent. You don't know what the issues are with the non-rebel. You see, at the extremes there are two ways for an adolescent to develop their identity: they can rebel (and we saw these above) or they can comply.

---

[37] BTW, I absolutely know when my kids read this, they will say I am . . . Hi kids! Thanks for reading my book.

Whilst boys and girls can adopt the compliant role, this is a pattern we more frequently see with girls, so please excuse the gendered language. As we discussed earlier (p. 103), girls are more sensitive to internalising the message of society about working hard, being nice, doing your best and then some. Many are uncomfortable with rebellion. Sometimes it is the quiet, compliant ones you have to watch.

I referred in the busyness business chapter to Taylor Swift's words about being trained to be happy if she got praise. These girls are often shaped in the childhood years. They suck up all the opportunities they are offered, ace the tasks of primary school. Even in early adolescence, they continue to thrive. They rote learn for their GCSEs and get a raft of top marks. But I often see them unravel in the more complex academic and social world of ages sixteen to eighteen, when they have to understand what they think themselves, rather than what is the socially approved answer, or when there starts to be ambiguity on what the right thing is to do. Life is more complex in late adolescence: school, parents, friends, the internet, love interests might all have clashing demands.

The outcome-based childhood puts kids on a path of stickers and star charts, of best-friend-forever necklaces, of 'be kind' T-shirts, of house points, merits, certificates, end-of-year awards. It trains them to stop looking internally at what they like and want and think, and rather, to always look externally at what is the right thing to do or what other people want. Their internal self is full of how they are not meeting the standards of the world – that they are 'only' getting an A, not an A*, or how they didn't get on this team or into that school. If you aim for perfect, there will always be a heap of ways you don't make the grade. They are so full of how they aren't good enough, they generally don't see themselves as perfectionists. In my book *The You Don't*

Understand Me Journal, I don't even use the word perfectionism, as so few teenagers connect with it. I call it 'best seeking'.

By the time girls like this get to adolescence, the wish to rebel or separate can be completely repressed; they fail to notice it at all. They have numbed their own wishes so successfully that the evolutionary drive to separate and individuate gets channelled into self-harm, academic 'perfection' or anorexia, without troubling their conscious mind at all. The predetermined good path is all: work hard, be kind.

Again, 'good girls' (who, remember, can also be boys) can present whatever your parenting style, but seems particularly fraught with a parent who holds on too tight. It can result with a spiralling up of standards, or in enmeshment and dependency: phoning or texting their parent over every decision and never risking the conflict that difference can create. With the parent who doesn't hold on tight enough, they can feel uncared for.

Either way, parents are often poleaxed by a daughter's mental illness. The signs were not there, and they come to clinic saying how she had always been amazing, beautiful, clever and never any trouble at all. I watch their daughter almost imperceptibly wince, as what her parents say with pride and joy is experienced by her as another expectation she has to meet. The trouble is kids need to be trouble. Humans are flawed and that needs to be allowed. We have trained a generation of girls, especially, to try to fit into everyone else's definition of perfect. They need to be encouraged to be themselves, to find their own individuality and risk the possible conflict that difference can involve.

THE CRAZY ADOLESCENCE BALANCING TRICK

The tricky bit for parents is balancing the holding on and letting go – the how and when of both – with your child's own natural style and psychology. It is the attachment dance again, except this time you are trying to co-ordinate your moves with someone who doesn't want to dance with you: you are watching, reacting, harmonising, but also sometimes changing the music. It is about staying firm, but also adapting and being flexible to who they are – and obviously these are contradictory demands. It seems like almost an impossible task. As I outlined at the beginning of the chapter, over these years, nearly every rule and boundary will have to change and yet you need to be as consistent as possible, and this is when your values can guide your path. You want to be letting the rope out at the right speed, so they are neither strangled by it nor drowning without it. You need to be constantly present and fade into the background as much as possible.

Over these years, you have to start to give up the firmness and the control, even if you don't want to and even if you don't think they are ready to meet your expectations. Clearly, you can't carry on being in charge when your child is twenty, twenty-five, thirty years old. It can help you let go, later on in adolescence, to give up the idea that *you know best* for this developing, future-fully-fledged adult. And that may be super hard. You may feel that you know *them* best; you knew them before they knew themselves – before they had the conscious notion of themselves. You also are so wise and understand how the world works. What do they know about career paths? Mortgages? Holding down a job?

But you need to accept there are lots of things that you don't know so well: it is hard to know anyone else's mind. We all get tens of thousands of thoughts a day, and how many of our teenage offspring's do we have access to? Or an adult child's? When you are teaching your baby to speak, you pay firm attention to try to articulate what they want. I was watching attentive parents in a café the other day, as their one-year-old cried and wailed and pointed, and they tried to guess what he wanted. By trial and error, they guessed it was a slice of watermelon that he saw at our table; then, once a slice was procured for him, he wanted to hold it himself but couldn't. Even deciphering simple thoughts like this is hard, but your teenager's thinking will be infinitely more complex, and they largely aren't motivated to share it. Unless they want something, obvs. Like Lana Del Rey tickets or new trainers; then, of course, you will hear about it straight away.

Their thinking is incredibly complex, fast-paced, and changes rapidly in the moment and over time. In therapy, when I am talking with an adolescent, sometimes I'll notice a shadow pass over their face – an almost imperceptible movement in a cheek or an eyebrow. And so I ask about it. We unpack that millisecond. And when we do, we discover they thought multiple different, sometimes contradictory things in that moment. They felt multi-layered emotions; it reminded them of many things from the past, and created a wish for the future. They were mindful of my thoughts, and many other people's. As parents, we tend to hold on to a version of our kids that has served us through time, and are reluctant to let go of it to acknowledge their new, more sophisticated cognitive landscape that we have very little access to. I will be talking about how to best stay in touch with it in the next chapter, but even then, you won't have a full understanding.

As they pass through adolescence, your children will have thoughts and opinions and ways of doing things that are nothing to do with you and probably nothing like you. You do have one very important perspective on them. But it is one that they may naturally react against as they establish what they think. Parents who give their opinion constantly risk infantilising their children, but often it is because they want to hold on to their own role and identity. However, when they do this, they are unwittingly tying their adolescent into always looking for that third-person validation. You may think, 'Well, I want them to care about my opinion, but just not other people's, not those people on Snapchat,' for example. But adolescents aren't wired like that: if you tie them into seeking validation from you, you tie them into seeking validation from the world in general. Instead, you need to help scaffold them into their own opinion, *which may be different from yours* (and in good news, the people on Snapchat's). As I said, it can be like a pendulum swing, with 'your way' at one end, and during adolescence 'their way' at the opposite one. Rest assured, at the end of this period of separation and individuation, you may find you both rest somewhere nearer the centre.

As parents, we tend to think we've done the hard work of establishing what we believe is 'the right way' through our own separation from the traditional values or routines of our parents. We feel our kids should recognise the 'rightness' of what we have established. If you have brought them up in a different culture than your culture of origin, this may be exacerbated. We dismiss our child's need to have just as many independent thoughts and wishes to do things differently as we did ourselves. It seems that we have raised our kids determined to give them every opportunity and chance we never had, and then we want them to totally agree with us and adopt our way of life. Fly, baby, fly . . . but just close to me, your parent.

For many of you, one of the hardest things you will do is let your almost-adult child have the autonomy they need to lead their own authentic life. The freedom to cock it up, make mistakes, get it wrong and learn from it, as you yourself did. But also the freedom to succeed on their own terms, without owing their success to your input. Many adolescents get that autonomy by fighting with you; others, our good girls and boys, may need a little loving push out of the nest. They may need you to go off on holiday without them, to not be so invested in their academic progress or to make your shopping trips with someone else. So that they have the freedom to do so, too.

All through this book I have been channelling the firm-but-kind message – the authoritative parent, who has plenty of control, rules and boundaries, but is also warm and supportive. It is in adolescence that you need to lose the firmness. You need to give them their freedom, and rely on maximising the kindness, the relationship and the warmth you have in the bank. In the next chapter, we will go for a last time to relationship, to look at how you do that.

4.3
Keeping Your Relationship Going

In these last chapters, we've covered the two important developmental tasks of adolescents, which are their need to form their own identity and to separate from you. We've discussed how to both avoid rebellion and to help them towards independence – you need to let go of firm and the belief you can control their outcome. Any influence or guidance you have with them as they reach the later years of adolescence should be through your relationship with them.

The trouble with that is that your relationship is likely to be at its lowest ebb. Back to our attachment-dance analogy: seemingly, they no longer want to dance with you as much. Oh, they might when they are in their tween years, with an air of embarrassment or duty, but as they go through the teenage years, less and less. They are off dancing in someone else's nightclub, and when they come back, somehow it feels as though *they* are setting the music, you don't quite get it, and you are dancing around them furtively, trying to find the moments when you are in sync.

Their urge towards separation and individuation from you can sometimes feel rude or brutal. You see them go and sit in the garden and you follow, ready for a chat and to spend some time with them, and they say, 'Why can't you leave me alone, for God's sake?' You pop into their bedroom in the evening to drop off some clean laundry, and they make 'yes' a three-syllable word, dripping with contempt. As their exposure to the outside world increases, as well as their capacity for abstract thought and hypothesis, they begin to question you and your beliefs. In doing so, they often become angry or disdainful of the world view, the habits and customs you have established. They may act like you have been keeping them in an odd cult where you do things in a particular way, and now they've seen the light, they wish to rebuff it all. In their disdain, they are not only rejecting you, but also their younger self who accepted living in your fiefdom without question.

Whilst we can know that this is normal in theory, in practice, it often feels deeply personal and wounding, like death by a thousand cuts. Everything you have worked for and all the sacrifices you have made – and now they are scoffing at you and rejecting you. It frequently evokes a 'he/she-is-so-ungrateful – don't-they-know-how-much-I-do-for-them' response in many parents. Including me. It's infuriating.

Many young people are not only 'rude' and 'ungrateful', but are also making a bit of a mess of stuff in some way: that can be making bad decisions with friends or romantically, with drugs or alcohol or in terms of school and their futures. They are almost certainly making a mess in their bedrooms. When they are being rejecting on the one hand and struggling on the other, you can oscillate between desperate worry and utter fury.

Many parents also feel that this is grossly different from 'our day', when we showed more respect to our parents. And it is true, that we, as a cohort of parents, have fostered these closer relationships, been much more involved in our children's lives and taken more of an interest in them. As a society, we have become less formal – not so long ago we were calling our friends' parents Mr and Mrs, and that now seems prehistoric. The way we dress, eat, behave, has become more casual. We have not only given them so much, we have also flattened the hierarchical relationship and therefore feel that we don't 'deserve' this backlash of rudeness, and that they should listen to us. Yet, it is also true that Shakespeare wrote: 'I would there were no age between ten and three-and-twenty, or that youth would sleep out the rest; for there is nothing in between but getting wenches with child, wronging the ancientry, stealing, fighting.' My point? That older generations have always been despairing of the disrespect teens show their elders.

When parents come to me with these different types and flavours of problems of worry or anger about their child, I listen and I try to understand. I meet with them, with and without their adolescent child. I try to understand the root of the problem (their beliefs and feelings), and I try to understand its expression (the self-harm, or the drugs, or the eating disorder). I try to understand from everyone's perspective. And when I have done all that, and I am thinking about how the parents can help, it more often than not comes down to one thing. My advice to them is this: try to hold on to your relationship with your adolescent.

Because as the direct supervision you have of them peters out, the amount of control you have over them fades. As they stop caring about your rules (unless they are a 'good girl', and then, as we have seen, they care too much) and feel the strong pull towards their peers and the start of their own generation, your influence in their life wanes. As I say, your relationship with them may be at its lowest ebb, but it's the best tool you've got for keeping them safe and on the manifesto pathway.

Of course, it might not be the only thing you need. If adolescents have serious mental-health issues or are acting unsafely, parents need to take charge in a more active way, including getting professional help, but your relationship is still of crucial importance.

There are other ways to keep your influence other than your relationship; I just don't recommend them. One is to try to keep your control through fear. If you over-value firm, you can end up being angry, threatening or fierce to try to scare them into submission in adolescence, but if you have a child of a rebellious bent, you will likely be forced into an escalation of punishment that you can never carry out. At an extreme, I'm sure some kids end up in care each year because of this sort of pattern. In a more compliant child, the 'good girl', it will likely lead to repression of themselves, into shame and anxiety.

Of course, their rudeness, lack of co-operation and unhelpfulness are exasperating, but this too-firm parenting is not a great way to try to keep your influence. It is a trap, and it is one that I too have sometimes fallen into. Their rudeness can trigger our own feelings of not being respected or listened to. These are painful feelings for nearly everyone, but also tap into times we've felt like this before – for example, in our jobs, relationships or family histories. It can evoke a feeling of 'God damn, if no one in the world listens to me, my kid is going to.' But you know the punchline before I tell you: of course, they are not. They are going to continue to rebel against you, whatever punishments you come up with – and then, they will eventually leave home.

The second way to keep your influence is through money, and perhaps we are all a little guilty here. We all use money as the sugar of influence over an older adolescent's life. It's natural and normal to have some sugar – but you don't want to be using it too much. They probably feel a pull away from you, but they know they can't afford the lifestyle they want. It is part of the social contract that you still support them financially, and have them live with you, through training or education, but it's a balance. Don't give them so much that they aren't motivated to get their butt out to work. And I don't just mean a career – I mean babysitting, waiting, shop work, whilst they are working towards their career. Nor so much that they can buy a shitload of drugs. When I meet parents who give their kids too much, it is generally unhelpful, but particularly when those kids aren't keeping their basic responsibilities – for example, going to school or helping at home. Being given a car when you are not keeping your basic responsibility is not a good lesson to learn.

I also meet some young people who seem scared to live their own lives for fear they won't be as successful or wealthy as their parents. That keeps them tied to their parents, for money or a lifestyle, in a really unhelpful way – often unconsciously resentful, but not actively rebellious. They end up holidaying with their parents in a five-star resort, despite the pull towards their friends who are camping in Wales.

Frequently using money to gain time with your child or influence when they should be off living their own life can be unhelpful. They need to experience the discomfort of not having the material goods or comfort that they are used to, as that will give them the drive to go and earn the money they need.

It's a hard balance to find with money, tbh. I wonder if the answer is giving them *nearly enough* allowance in teenage years ... enough that they can join in amongst their peers, but not so much that they get into a heap of trouble or get used to a standard of living they cannot support themselves. Nearly enough might keep them that bit keener to make friends with you after the fight, to do the chores and to generally be a bit pleasanter. You neither want them to be overcome by frugality or guilt about money, nor a profligate spender of your cash (or spoilt, as we used to call it). But nor do you want to be resentful that, despite you giving them every material good they want, they are rude to you. Being rude to you is par for the course, and you can't buy your way out of it. I would try to avoid getting into monetising everything – every daily chore and every bit of compliance – but that doesn't mean you can't pay them to do a big weekly job, like the ironing or mowing the lawn. I would also try to avoid using money as a threat or a bribe. Try to give what you give freely without resentment.

But fear and money aside, the most important influence you have over your kiddult is your relationship with them. From eleven, you are moving along the control continuum from where you have almost total control, to eighteen, where you have almost none, and the thing that keeps kids on the straight and narrow and gives them the best chance of good mental health is a strong relationship with their parents.

Because when they find themselves at 2am drunk, wearing one shoe and with someone dodgy offering them a lift home, you want them to call you. Well, you do and you don't want them to call you, but overall you do. You don't want your kid making daft, potentially life-changing decisions, without your influence. And if your influence is only through fear or money, they might make the wrong one. But a strong sense of you, your care in their life, will help them make the right safe decision in that moment. Even if they slammed the door and told you they hated you this morning.

I'm going to introduce a new analogy for you to help you with your parenting in adolescence. You need to be like the central heating in their life: largely ignored, but ready in the background to be warm when needed. Usually there, adolescents only really notice central-heating parenting when it is not working – when it is cold and then they moan and bitch about it. When it is working, it is totally ignored and taken for granted, which – as we discussed earlier – is the flip side of unconditional love. To be warm and in the background, you need to let go of a whole heap of stuff; watch and listen in on their life, avoid advice and parent by example. Let's look at these in more detail.

LETTING GO OF STUFF
I see a lot of young people in my clinic who are self-harming, and in the first appointment I generally see them with their parents. Sometimes they are the good-girl type whose parents praise their compliance, and as they do so, I watch the girl sink lower in her chair into the self-hatred that repressed emotion through compliance brings. But others are less compliant, and then the conversation often goes like this: their parents are desperately worried about their self-harm, but also about their attitude generally. They are rude, they are not applying themselves properly in school, their outfits are terrible (often skimpy/sexy), they are vaping/smoking/smoking weed, they are out all hours and their rooms are a mess.

In my sessions, I do try to be genuinely compassionate and understand the parents' point of view, but I just want a reality check here. Half those things don't belong on that list. If your child is so miserable and/or anxious that they are self-harming, not eating or having panic attacks, the main things that should be on your list of concerns are their thoughts and feelings. Thoughts and feelings are the nuts and bolts of mental health, and if your child is behaving in a self-harming/not-eating/panic-attack kind of way, we can be pretty sure that there is something wrong with their mental health. Their thoughts and feelings are what need to be on your list of concerns. *Try to let go of everything else.*

All of us as parents can learn something from this. And it is this: I have never heard a case of a parent nagging a child that has resulted in them turning over a new leaf and changing from a messy person to a tidy person. Indeed, I would wager that as a topic it tops the league for disconnection between 'so much time, energy and angst put in in adolescent years' vs 'amount of genuine change got out'. It is ironic because it is one of those factors that generally resolves itself – messy young people normally grow into relatively tidy middle-aged people. Well, it either resolves, or they leave and then it's not your problem anymore. In my own home, I found rooms suddenly got very tidy and personal hygiene drastically improved when a romantic interest was visiting. Problem solved.[38]

I have had this conversation a lot with parents, and most of them have genuinely believed that I just don't understand how awful their child's room is – so much worse than any other child's. They try to convince me, that if I knew, then I'd understand. The parents sometimes go on to tell me that their child is doing harm to the room in some way (for example, nail-varnish-remover pads on the carpet, or mould growing), and yes, this is where I draw the line on intervention, both generally and on rooms. If their mess, or whatever it is, is doing genuine harm to some of your property or to someone else, then you get to intervene. And no, I don't mean offending-your-sensibilities harm, I mean actual harm. But even then, I would often let it go.

---

[38] There are new problems caused when a romantic interest visits, tbh. Swings and roundabouts.

Why? Because it's not effective, and you have limited cards to play in your relationship with your teen before you run out of relationship with them, so why play one on something ineffective? It's like betting on the horse with three legs. Save your bet for something worthwhile that is going to matter.

Ditto vaping and smoking. I think you are well within your rights to lay down the law a bit with a younger child on this, but as they get to fifteen or sixteen, how effective is it going to be? I think this is a rare one where you might want to curtail the monetary allowance, as that is a logical consequence. That might look like, without anger or rancour: 'I don't want to pay for your e-cigarettes, so I'm taking £5 off your monthly allowance'. But tbh, if they are determined to smoke or vape, they will find a way, including doing something iffy or illegal to get it.

Getting involved with how a growing teen dresses is also difficult. This is often gendered, as parents worry that girls' sexualised dress sends out the wrong message or puts them at risk of attack. This is sometimes at odds with a belief that women and girls should be able to dress however they want without risk of attack. Personally, I think we are on dodgy ground here of teaching girls to monitor their own behaviour, rather than putting the responsibility on men and boys. However, I think we can try to teach them about the appropriateness of dress – for example, is a sexy outfit appropriate for a job interview? I also worry about the self-objectification – i.e. fitting themselves into a sexualised image largely created by men, which distances them from finding their own sexy. However, in terms of influence, we have very little. We know that anything we say will be ignored and if we really get hardline about it, they will hide the sexy outfit in their bag to change into later. As my mother did in the Sixties with her new, skin-tight jeans before my granny found and burned them.

On top of the practical stuff, there are a whole heap of things about how your adolescent treats you, which you shouldn't let go of completely, but are best not taken too personally, including compliance, respect, expecting the truth and politeness. Adolescents are often rude, non-compliant and disrespectful to their parents: they don't answer; they answer back; they tell you that you are unreasonable; they poke holes in your arguments; expect everything; give nothing. If they are not doing this, they may be suppressing the urge and trying to people-please, or, unconsciously, they may not be confident enough in your love to be rude, or in your strength to take their rebellion.

It is also normal for teenagers to lie: research indicates that 95 per cent of teenagers lie to their parents, and the scientist who did this research jokes that the others might be lying to researchers![cvii] But if it's any consolation, the main reason they lie is that they don't want to upset their parents. The main type of lie is avoidance of discussing the issue or, if forced to talk about it, just leaving out part of the story.

On a recent holiday, when I was clashing a lot with one of mine, in the escalating 'don't-be-so-rude; don't-speak-to-me-like-that' vein, I set myself a reminder on my phone every day: it's not personal; let it go. That allowed me to breathe, say calmly, 'I don't like it when you speak to me like that' and move on with the day. Without my arguing with them, we didn't get into the pointless escalation about whether or not they had been rude, or whether I'd been rude first, etc. The whole thing went much better; they behaved better. I'd set an expectation on behaviour, but I stopped expecting immediate compliance: I am not expecting them not to act as a teenager when they are one. I am expecting that this is a standard they will grow into in their life.

Maybe you think I'm being 'too kind', not firm enough? Perhaps. I just never see firm-firm work that well with teenagers, i.e. the direct confrontation or keeping strict rules. The firm that is shown to work, in my opinion as well as the research, is that based on mutual respect, trust and expecting them to make mistakes. It is a firmness set on repetition of boundaries, on being kind, using humour and warmth to dissipate and being in a war of attrition, rather than escalation to win on this. I gave an example of how this might play out in the last chapter – setting a boundary, it being mildly broken, resetting the boundary without getting drawn into an argument or an arms race of punishment. Repeat. Repeat. Repeat. Again, as I've said before, compliance on behaviour amongst teenagers may be poor, but absorption of parents' values is high.

And the main reason to let go of most of those things? Because they get in the way of the most important thing, which is maintaining your relationship with them. Value your relationship with them more than compliance – both are possible, but just as kind trumps firm, so relationship trumps compliance. And what else do you need to maintain that? You watch and listen, with empathy and curiosity, from the position of having your own life. More on your own life later, but for now, watching and listening . . .

WATCHING AND LISTENING OUT
So as the central heating in your kid's life, you need to be self-adjusting the warmth you are putting out all the time. You are monitoring their temperature, and in reality that means a lot of watching and listening. It means creating a lot of time when you are together, and staying warm, avoiding advice. You need to be both frequently present and fade into the background.

You need your own life, so that you don't resent this largely passive position.

Personally, I swear by the family meal. In my home, we usually eat together. It is not *The Waltons*. Often, it does my head in. The bickering, the table manners, the ingratitude for the meal and the lack of consideration of me as a person. But it does allow me to watch and listen: to hear in some way about their days; to see and feel their moods; to have some idea of what is going on in their lives. I hope it gives them some sense of family.

The kitchen around bedtime is another good place to watch and listen, as the teenager prowls around for a late-night snack. Or a regular trip to drop off laundry whilst they are in their room can be useful. Their friends coming round is also excellent stalking ground for the watching-and-listening parent. You don't want to be the parent trying to get down with the kids, but you do want to try to connect with their friends a bit, being friendly and easy-going, providing a space if you can, and snacks. And every parent of a teenager's favourite: the car lift. Perfect, in that they are contained, stuck with you, and a little bit reliant and grateful, with no eye contact. Even better if you also give their friend(s) a lift: they will almost forget you are there, like an anonymous taxi driver, and you will squirrel away whatever information you glean.

This sounds a bit calculated, and I don't mean it to be. You might ask what are you watching and listening for? You are watching and listening for an insight into their life and times. You are no longer the expert on your child. They are forming bonds with their peers, having interests, creating language, demarcating their generation – a place that is always going to be a foreign land to you. This is the place where your child will live, and you, by definition, can only be a visitor to it. But your child is part of it, and you should try to understand it, to understand them, to foster your relationship with them and to be aware of the dangers that lie there.

Believe me, I have been a therapist to hundreds of adolescents: the things that you are watching for are more than the messy bedroom; these are heartbreaking things like being rejected and left out by people you trusted and thought cared for you; these are being assaulted by someone you thought you loved; these are a secret awful thing they did once that they've never told anyone about; these are a fear that they are uniquely hideous and awful and no one will ever love them, or terror that they will never succeed or get a job. These are the extremely painful feelings of not being enough, not being good enough, that might result in your child being anxious, depressed or disenfranchised, or in trying to numb those feelings with drugs, not eating, porn or self-harm. So you, their parent, are not sweating the small stuff, watching and listening, as this is your best attempt at understanding this person who inhabits a different generation from you, who you don't know so well anymore. You are watching and listening for those hints of problems, ready with your warmth, hoping they will talk to you if there is a problem. And then what? Well, then you try to talk to them by really listening.

REALLY LISTENING
Really listening to your kids is hard work and likely goes against all your natural instincts. I call the listening parents normally do 'parent-pause listening'. Parent-pause listening is where we listen to our kids up to the first time they pause, and then we jump in to tell them what to do. Parent-pause listening and its near cousin, 'the giving of unsolicited advice', are two of the

main reasons teenagers don't talk to their parents. We are inadvertently damaging our relationship with our teenager when we listen like this.

Why 'telling people what to do' has not become extinct from an evolutionary point of view, I don't know. We all hate it. I am fifty-four and it still evokes a feeling in me that I want to do completely the opposite of what I am told. The more compliant kids, the 'good girls', may do it, but inside it is turned to self-hatred. The less compliant kids just do exactly the opposite. Why do we persist?

Because do you know what none of the teenagers I've seen in therapy have ever said to me? It is this: 'I wish my parents gave me more advice'. Indeed, thinking about it now, none of my adult patients has ever said this to me either. In fact, have the words ever been spoken by anyone in the history of humanity? Is anyone crying out for more advice from their parents? Unsolicited advice is just criticism in a different form.

This always reminds me of the 1992 pop psychology book *Men Are from Mars, Women Are from Venus*. Did you read it? Its premise, in two sentences, was this: when women have problems they want to talk to their men about them, and when they do, men try to solve their problems. Women don't want their problems solved, they want to talk them over and be listened to.

As kids, I don't think we talked much to our parents about our problems; they were too busy having their own lives. Today's children do talk to us more, I think, and generally I think this is a positive thing, but when they do, *they generally do not want those problems solved.* They, like the rest of us in a fractured world, want to be heard and understood. They want someone who actively listens to them, lets them mull things over and come to a solution themselves. You don't have to agree; you just have to 'get' them. This is part of letting them learn to be their own adult and having a decent relationship with them as that adult. Indeed, I would argue that you may not be in a position to solve their problems, as you don't live in their generation.

But this active listening. I think you can do that. Your two tools: empathy and curiosity. Remember these from Chapter 3.3, 'Relationships in childhood': your mental-health first-aid kit. Your trusty go-tos. You reach for them any time they need to 'talk', and by 'talk' I mean, listen.

So just to be clear what I mean by empathy. I mean really trying to understand how they are thinking and feeling. There's a moment sometimes in therapy where a young person pauses, struggles to find the word they are looking for, trying to describe an abstract psychological experience, and I find myself finishing their sentence. And they look at me and say, 'Yes, that's it.' And I think, 'I've got this person well enough. I'm sufficiently in their way of thinking and looking at the world that I can finish their sentence.' And generally, I find that a pretty good predictor of outcome. My first book for teenagers was called *You Don't Understand Me* for a reason, and that reason is that the feeling of being misunderstood is endemic, and the power of being understood incredible.

To get there you need curiosity. And to get curiosity you have to let go of two more things: the idea that you know your adolescent better than they know themselves and the idea that you know best. You *knew* them best, but they grew up and they have hundreds of interactions and thousands of thoughts every day that you know nothing about. Ask. When you get the opportunity, ask. Ask open questions, without judgment, without any agenda except empathy.

Sometimes, *they say they do want you to solve the problem*, and here we need to think about both what is actually helpful and what is developmentally appropriate. Again, in the childhood relationships chapter, I warned against intervening in friendship dilemmas, which is rarely effective in my experience. As they get older, solving the problem is often a poisoned chalice. Of course, part of your adolescent wants to be a child – don't we all at times? Don't we all want someone to wrap us up and take us in their arms and make everything OK again? On the other hand, the evolutionary drive in them is separation and individuation, and so when you try to solve, you will likely be wrong both in their mind, and in reality, too, as you don't live in their shoes, in their generation, and really don't know best. In a way, though, if by some fluke you chance upon a good solution, you are 'right', and this opens a different set of problems: you are undermining their autonomy; you may be infantilising them or keeping them dependent on you. I would argue that it is potentially better that they make the wrong decision by themselves than for you to make the right decision for them.

Which isn't to say that you don't support and scaffold them: you listen, you try to understand, you are curious. They are often looking for the emotional dump, where they offload all their worries on you, and then sail forth unencumbered. Or they are looking for you to agree with them; the reassurance of having you to blame if it then goes wrong. You may need to say the magic words 'Do you want my advice on this? Or are you just looking to talk it through?' and if the answer is that they don't want your advice, you zip it. If they do want your advice, offer it tentatively: it could be right or could be wrong advice.

Our adolescent kids, if we have kept a semblance of a relationship going, will likely contact us far more than we contacted our parents. We've trained them with all our star charts, learning objectives and all adult-led busyness activities to look for the opinion of others, and then given them the ideal means to seek it out in the mobile phone. It's a perfect storm to make them dependent on us. They tempt us all the time to advise, to solve, to step in, but us doing so paralyses them in making their own mistakes and owning their own lives.

APOLOGISING
In this book, I have come back again and again to the concept of being good enough and not aiming for perfection, and the main reason I have done this is because of the example it sets to your children. Again, I say, they do not put their shoes on when you ask, but they absorb your values. The values of good enough – balance, acceptance, compassion, forgiveness; these are the values of good mental health.

There's one more important thing. Sometimes, when I give a talk to parents at a school or such like, I get asked about whether you should apologise to your kids. It always surprises me: there are few simple answers in adolescent psychology, but this one is so easy. Yes, emphatically, yes. Why wouldn't we apologise? I also hear from young people a lot that their parents never apologise. Perhaps their parents want to keep an illusion of being consistently right or powerful – a perfect parent – never wrong. I recognise this feeling – I had it in my pursuit of time out with my toddler and I was wrong then, and it is certainly wrong with an infinitely more psychologically complex teenager. Sometimes parents seem to think that they will lose control if they apologise; perhaps similar to how they feel about child-led play – that anarchy will take over if they let the control slip for one moment. Perhaps they actually believe that they are perfect, or they always know best. Or perhaps they fear using their own vulnerability in their parenting.

But, of course, we aren't perfect, and we don't know best about everything, and we should be teaching by example, which is the most powerful teaching of all. In the good-enough life, we accept that we all make mistakes all the time, and are prepared to reflect on that and consider the feelings of others. Vulnerability is necessary for true relationships. Let me say this again: if you want to have a true relationship with your adult child, some of that will be about your own vulnerability; your willingness to learn from them, to own up and to say sorry when necessary. If you are not apologising, you are gaslighting them into your manipulated reality where you didn't cock up. This is terrible for your relationship with them – you will lose their respect by not apologising; but denying the reality that you ever make mistakes is also terrible for their mental health.

So yes, I apologise. In fact, I apologise all the frigging time. I apologise much more than anyone else in the house. Oh, sorry, I'm running late. Sorry, the milk was off. I know you don't love this meal, but it was the best I can do, sorry. I'm sorry I can't drive you, I'm working. I'm sorry, that was a mean thing to say, I didn't mean it. I'm sorry I left the room, I was losing it and I needed to calm down. And of course, sorry, I lost it. Sorry for shouting. Again.

I apologise to set the example that being wrong, making mistakes and making amends are an intrinsic part of the human position. If we never apologise, how are they going to learn how to apologise to their friends, their partner, their work colleagues? They are going to associate apologising with the forced apology of a parent chastising a child, or the shame-filled apology of being a bad person. Apologising is the rebuttal of the perfection position – it allows imperfection and accepts it as a normal part of life. We need to teach kids how to be wrong, to learn, to grow, and we teach that not with spiralling arguments, but by demonstrating how to be imperfect, with grace and compassion, ourselves. It also demonstrates the emotional competence that we are looking for – the capacity to bear complex situations where mistakes are made.

INTERVENING

Inevitably, as a central-heating parent, you will need to turn the warmth up at times. They will stumble. You may notice, or they may come and tell you. I believe they will come and tell you more if you haven't been telling them how to micro-manage their life, and if you are honest with your own mistakes.

You are watching and listening in the background of their life, as, when things go wrong for them, sometimes you may need to intervene. You may need your firm-and-kind and relationship-based parenting to find a way to help them. Some young people will require professional help. That can be hard for a parent, as they want their child to talk to them, but of course, the neutrality a professional offers can never be replicated in a parent. As a parent, you simply feel their pain more, and that makes it difficult for them to tell you things in full, and for you to offer the more detached space of the professional. Believe me, I can't offer my own children the calm, wise space I offer my patients.

Sometimes, with some of the most serious mental illnesses, such as anorexia, drug addiction or suicidality, parents have to take up a more active parenting role. Mental illness is sometimes a regression to an earlier time of life, where they re-need the consistency of boundaries to help keep themselves safe. You may have to flex your firm muscles again to make them eat; to keep them away from danger. But firmness is not for when they are not making the grade or wearing what you want. Firmness like that is only for the emergencies – don't use it up on untidy rooms.

BY EIGHTEEN

So we draw the adolescent section to a close. What do I want you to know, and where do you want to be?

As your kid hits their eighteenth birthday, they may be starting to prepare for a post-school life, where they may go off to college or university at the other end of the country; travel or go into the workforce, expected to be as adult as everyone else. But many will still be in a state of flux; not knowing what to do next, or what to do given their exam results. Emotions are still running high at this age – brain development continues into the early twenties – and the changes that the end of school brings can be scary or overwhelming to them. They don't magically turn into rational adults at the point they gain legal responsibility.

Largely, you should treat them as though they have. Act into the change you want to see. Check your own feelings; your sadness at losing them can warp your assessment of their capacity to cope. Too often, I hear parents justify their own interventions on the basis of their child's immaturity. Chicken and egg, I reckon. Your jumping in to solve, quicker, more efficiently and more knowledgeably, will block their inevitably more clumsy efforts. Let them take care of themselves a bit more and solve their own problems when they can. Let them cook inedible food, shrink stuff in the washing machine, burn their nose when they don't wear sunscreen, and oversleep and annoy their friends by being late. Don't say 'I told you so'. Then they'll learn those lessons for themselves and act with self-motivation, rather than the resentment of being told.

Few parents feel their work is done at this age, but your work should be increasingly more on the sidelines. Hopefully, you feel that you've set the foundations for future good mental health, even if they are struggling now. We would hope for some signs of joy, a capacity to bear the uncertain without paralysing anxiety, some belief that they are good enough and have something to offer the world.

Maybe they talk to you; maybe they don't. This, I think, has as much to do with their own personality as yours: some kids are not talkers. It's hard to grow a tropical plant in an English summer – but you can do your best to provide the optimal conditions. But they will likely never come to you opening up if you just think you know best, use it as opportunity to say, 'I told you so' and tell them what to do. I mean, would you open up with someone like that?

We over-advise and over-intervene, despite our memories of how annoying that was when our own parents did it. We rationalise it by believing we are oh so different from them. We are woke, trendy, down with the kids. We are interested in them, not like our own parents. We want to help. We understand the modern world. But, not to our kids we don't. To our kids, we will always be from the past – a different place. We will always be Dad/Mum-dancing and slightly embarrassing. We will always be staid and sensible. But our kids sometimes want staid and sensible. They want to pass their ideas around with someone who will treat them respectfully and warmly. Their good-enough, kind, relationship-based parent.

4.4
You, as a Parent with Adolescent and Adult Children

I wanted to bookend my book with chapters about you as a parent. We had a chapter in Part 1, thinking about you becoming a parent, and here we are at the other end, thinking about you as the parent of an emerging adult. This will likely involve you setting down your parenting reins, for large chunks of your days and weeks. You will likely never rid yourself of them completely – once a parent, always a parent – but you just shouldn't be using them that much anymore. I wrote in that first chapter that parenting was a marathon that lasted the rest of your life, but as your child becomes legally an adult the intensity of this should fade away. It's not that you stop caring, stop loving or stop worrying completely, but physically, you (should) have less to do. You should have time to breathe.

I've given you my framework for parenting, of being good enough, relationship-based and firm and kind, and we've seen how in the adolescent years, it becomes more about the relationship than anything else. We've seen how, especially in the second half of the adolescent years, you letting go is key to your child stepping into their life and having the autonomy to make their own decisions without feeling your influence. That includes your passive influence: no pursed lips or rolled eyes or, 'Well, you know what I think' with a disapproving face. It's also about you turning off Find My Phone or Microsoft-365 and letting them step into their freedom. It is about you really believing that you have been a good-enough parent and have raised a young adult capable of making the decision to have a life that's nothing like yours. It's about allowing your child to be who they are, and you being OK with that. Not just acting OK – they know you so well; they are exquisitely tuned in to what you are not saying, and they will see through any bullshit – but actually being OK. That is your challenge.

You have to let go of their outcome: failure and backward steps are a part of every story. It is hard to think of any adult I know whose life has been a straight trajectory of upward success, and yet we collude in society by selling kids that dream. As a parent, you need to be allowing and preparing for them to have a zig-zag education/career/life path, which allows them to change and develop, and find their own place. If you can, to paraphrase Rudyard Kipling, meet your child's triumph and disasters with equanimity: you are only invested in their wellbeing for them, not you, and you don't believe that it is inextricably linked to their academic achievement, appearance or outward expressions of success. You are proud of them as a person, not what they achieve. You are proud of your relationship with them.

Throughout the book, the issue of parenting by example comes back again and again; of you being the change you want to see. On the practical things, like phone use, eating and apologising, and on the abstract things like compromise, flexibility and tolerating imperfection and uncertainty. This parenting by example should extend to the whole manifesto. My manifesto for mental health is for you, too, not just your children. As your adolescent or young adult begins to separate from you, that is particularly important, as by taking care of yourself you allow them to move to adulthood. Let's think about those six keystones in relation to you.

You will inevitably be ageing, facing the major changes in your life as your kids grow up and potentially leave home, and perhaps facing your parents needing your help, too, or maybe their deaths. You will be likely facing the limitations on your own life: your successes, failures, ups and downs of life. How can you feel good enough? How can you meet yourself with the compassion you need to accept the less-than-perfect life you've achieved? And how can you meet the mistakes you've made as a parent with the wisdom of retrospect? It is rare that a parent gets their sense of self-esteem from their adolescent or adult child. When they were a baby, they demanded you with a ferocious cry, and now they likely need to push you away with the same ferocity. Sometimes mean or unkind, often thoughtless, as they step into adulthood, they will likely have little brain capacity to think about things from your perspective. There is a whole world of opportunity out there to figure out. Why would they be thinking about the central heating if it's working fine? You are, remember, the background on their life.

So what will give you joy in this part of your life? How can you fill the hours previously spent matching socks and emptying the dishwasher with something you love? My mother, legend that she is, took up tap dancing and trampolining as I left home. What an example that was to me, that being a grown-up was going to be OK. But laying down your anxiety is important, too. Of course, you will worry about them at times, but you can't be worrying about them all the time;

they shouldn't dominate your thoughts. If they do, you need to find something else to do: something you love, or something that matters, or something that is bigger than you and them. I warned you of this at the start: you need your own life – because that gives them freedom to have theirs. Can you embrace a new selfishness or laziness that gives them agency over their own life? I know you may feel sad losing this role that gave you so much joy and a sense of control and importance but losing this role you should be. You want them to have the pride of achieving things for themselves, rather than always feeling it was linked to parental support.

I often sense that parents (particularly mums) see or express worry almost as a sign of caring. I think that might be our old nemesis: how-I-want-to-be-seen. The oh-so-caring mother, so giving, so revered, so selfless – no thoughts for herself, but only for her children. I can fall for this trope myself. Let me be clear: our worry (my worry) is not a gift for our children. Indeed, I hope you have seen through this book that anxiety is toxic in parent–child relationships: it can be contagious or controlling, but in this kiddult stage of life, as they start to leave home, it can mean that they will avoid you. If they know you are going to worry or make a fuss, they simply won't tell you. I often see cycles of secrecy in families, where no one is telling anyone else anything. Or worse, when talking happens, but only behind each other's backs, and no one is talking directly, for fear of worrying each other. Aaaarggghhh! This sort of secrecy will undermine a good-enough relationship with your adultish kid.

You want to be aiming for some degree of emotional competence yourself. The capacity to self-reflect, to name and own what you feel, to take responsibility for it, whilst still valuing and being kind to yourself. There are strong emotions associated with this stage of life: regret, rejection, loss, loneliness (as well as perhaps a growing sense of freedom or opportunity); coming to terms with these in yourself is likely to be necessary if they are not going to pollute your relationship with your child. Your kids are not responsible for your emotional wellbeing. There is a thin line between the positive thing of you being emotionally vulnerable, honest and open about mistakes with them, as discussed in the last chapter, and, on the other hand, the less desirable situation of you emotionally dumping on them. That line is sustained by your own responsibility for your emotions.

Your relationship with them will also ideally involve you being as independent and capable as you can, including trying to not be dependent on them for your happiness. Of course, you want to see them, but your wellbeing should not be wholly taken up by your need for them to call or visit. One of the hardest parts of parenting an adult is the not knowing things and the not interfering. As your children start to change into adults, use your friendships as a guide of what you should and shouldn't ask about: do you ask your friends if they've been to the dentist recently? Or tell them, unsolicited, what you think of their outfit or partner? Do you tell them they are paying too much money on rent? No, you do not. Yes, the parent–adult child relationship is different to a friendship; I'm not saying it's exactly the same, as you still likely give them much more than you give your friends. All I'm saying is that one of the things you shouldn't give is your advice. Unsolicited advice is just criticism, remember? Your adult child has the right to let their teeth rot, wear whatever they want and date an idiot. Like you did. You will be far less annoying to them, and likely your relationship will be better, if you mind your own business. They are not your business anymore – they've started a new company.

This manifesto item, of your independence, can be a double-edged sword for parents, as it is sometimes resisted by kids. Adolescents and young adults can be, I find, keen to objectify you into the role of parent when it suits them: you taking care of them and maintaining the family home for them to opt in and out of as they wish. Your children may treat you, literally and metaphorically, like an all-they-can-eat buffet – rejecting most of you but taking more than they need of what they want. You are under no obligation to provide either of these buffets, of course, and not providing them will do them no harm. Whilst a parent–child relationship is nearly always one-sided, with you likely picking up the cheque, being the dumping ground for emotional angst and the cook/clothes washer/driver, you should definitely not feel like you always have to be there 24/7, as was more important when they were little. Indeed, the opposite should be true: you should try not to be always there, breaking their stereotype of you as a parent, and giving them their freedom as you take your own.

They may change the boundaries regularly: they may emotionally dump on you one day and then not want to talk about it the next. Indeed, they will often feel embarrassed after such an emotional dump, then pull away from you more the next day, to re-establish the boundary. That is what it means to be the parent of an adult child. Yes, I agree it's not fair. It is, however, your lot.

Every relationship involves compromise, and your job is to get on with this person, your grown child you didn't choose and can't control. You shaped and nurtured them, but likely that didn't turn out quite as you planned and is possibly more in line with Newton's third law of motion: 'for every action (force) there is an equal and opposite reaction'. They may react against your way of doing things, particularly if you are interfering, but give them the space they need as they start to establish their adult life according to their standards, not yours, and they will likely ping back towards you in time.

Being the parent of a nearly adult can be a retreat back to an earlier time, when you didn't have them as a responsibility, or it can be a new path to grow in a different direction. I made an analogy of being a central-heating parent earlier – in the background, providing regular warmth. But I'd just like to point out that central heating doesn't run itself: it requires regular maintenance and servicing, and somebody needs to pay for the fuel, and this is true of you, too. Somebody needs to take care of you, and that somebody is likely you. Your young-adult children are unlikely to do this for you, and nor should you expect them to, as they start on figuring out their own independent lives. You need to look after you, and that is for their benefit, as well as for yours.

As night follows day, the cycles of life turn. As a parent, you gave yourself to their love and now capitulate to the loss, as you gracefully accept an honourable retreat. You do so hopefully cognisant of having offered them a good-enough childhood, mindful of your mistakes, but knowing that perfection is a myth designed by ad agencies. Firm, now irrelevant, your power waned, but a good-enough relationship hopefully the legacy of your parenting.

ACKNOWLEDGEMENTS

Thanks go to my friend and colleague Cynthia Rousso, who constantly challenges me to both do better and accept my imperfections. I appreciate you always reading my work before I inflict it on anyone else; but more, I appreciate our mutual supervision and discussions of all aspects of mental health, parenting, education, personal growth. These have been key in developing my clinical practice and my thinking.

Thank you, Nick. You were there when I started planning this book and since then, you have offered me support nearly every day, listening to me empathically whilst I droned on. You have inspired me through your fortitude, patience and kindness. Thank you, too, for being one of my first readers and for your insightful, honest feedback, and also for the excellent central-heating analogy.

Thank you to Sarah Harrison for your parenting support over the years, and joining me in the messy middle of parenting indecision and meandering. Thank you for reading this in an early draft and giving me confidence to carry on. Thanks to Richard Ambrose for his advice from the frontier of middle-childhood boys. Thank you to Lucy Serpell, too, for reading the draft, and for your helpful comments. Sorry to Rach, Tash, Becky and Annie for missing our reunion as I approached my book deadline.

Thank you to Angela Rigg, who helped me keep my clinical work organised whilst I was writing this book. Also to Emma Nelson, who kindly gave me media training after I wrote my first book, and was flailing around about what to say to journalists.

Thanks go to my professional team: to my agent, Victoria Hobbs, for your care and clear-sightedness. To Carolyn Thorne and Susannah Otter, editors at Yellow Kite, for your enthusiasm. You made me believe I had something useful to say. Thank you to Anne Newman for editing my repetitions, rants and non-sequiturs so judiciously. I have tried my best to represent the research and my experience as accurately and helpfully as possible. However, I am sure mistakes remain, which of course, are my responsibility and for which I apologise in advance.

Thank you to all my current and former patients and their families, for being brave enough to come to therapy and share your stories. This book is, of course, inspired by you. I learnt so much from you, and I hope it helps you.

I have been blessed in life with a happy childhood and wonderful kids. I thank my dad, sadly no longer with us, and mum for never putting any pressure on me, and being vaguely amazed and very proud when I achieved anything, without any further expectation. As I say, a good attachment is the ultimate heirloom; I had that, and I hope I've passed it on.

So most of all, thank you to my three kids, Joe, Ella and Charlie: thank you for teaching me most of what I know about parenting. Thank you, too, for letting me mine your childhood to share these stories and illustrate ideas. It's been a blast being your mum: I'm pretty sure I haven't been perfect; I hope I've been good enough.

References

i   Brown, B. (2021), *Atlas of the Heart*. Vermilion.
ii Winnicott, D.W. (1953), 'Transitional Objects and Transitional Phenomena'. *Int. J. Psycho-Anal*, 34; 89–97. For an easier introduction to Winnicott's work, I would suggest Winnicott, D.W. (1964), *The Child, the Family and the Outside World*. Pelican Books. Or Phillips, A. (1997), *Winnicott*: Fontana Modern Masters.
iii Cecil, C.A., et al. (2017), 'Disentangling the mental health impact of childhood abuse and neglect'. *Child Abuse and Neglect*, 63, 106–19.
iv Bomback, A. (2022), 'How Economic Anxiety and Demographic Changes turned "parent" into a verb'. *KQED*.
v   Bull, Andy (2019), 'Jonny Wilkinson: "It took a few years for the pressure to really build. And then it exploded"' *The Guardian*, Monday 9th Sept.
vi Egan, S.J., Wade, T.D. and Shafran, R. (2011), 'Perfectionism as a transdiagnostic process: a clinical review'. *Clin Psychol Rev*, 31; 203–12.
vii Flett, G.L., Hewitt, P.L. Oliver, J.M. and McDonald, S. (2002), 'Perfectionism in Children and their Parents: A Developmental Analysis'. In G.L. Flett & L. Hewitt (Eds.) *Perfectionism: Theory, research, and treatment* (pp.89–132). Washington, DC: American Psychological Association.
viii For all things Mo, see https://www.mogawdat.com
ix Jung, C. (1981) Collected Works, Vol 17, The Development of Personality. Princeton University Press.
x   Julian, M.M. (2013), 'Age at adoption from institutional care as a window into the lasting effects of early experience'. *Clin. Child Fam Psychol Rev*, 16 (2) 101–45.

REFERENCES

xi May, K. (2018), p.245, *The Electricity of Every Living Thing*. Trapeze.

xii Baumrind, D. (1967), 'Child care practices anteceding three patterns of preschool behavior'. *Genetic Psychology Monographs*, 75(1), 43–88.

xiii Smetana, J.G., (2017), 'Current Research on parenting styles, dimensions, and beliefs'. *Current Opinion in Psychology*, 15, 19–25.

xiv Oster, E. (2019), *Cribsheet*: Penguin Press.

xv https://data.worldbank.org/indicator/SE.TER.ENRR.FE?end=2022&start=1970&view=chart

xvi Bolton, P. (2012), 'Education: Historical Statistics – House of Commons Library Standard Note SN/SG/4252.pdf.

xvii Bolton, P. (2024), Higher education student numbers. House of Commons Library

xviii Warren, E. and Warren-Tyagi, A. (2004), *The Two Income Trap. Why Middle Class Parents are Going Broke.* Basic Books.

xix Geoffroy, M., Cote, S.M., Parent, S. and Seguin, J.R. (2006), 'Daycare attendance, stress and mental health'. *Can. J. Psychiatry*, 51 (9).

xx Lowe Vandell, D., Burchinal, M. and Pierce, K.M. (2016), 'Early child care and adolescent functioning at the end of high school: Results from the NICHD Studies of Early Child Care and Youth Development'. *Developmental Psychology*, 52 (10), 1634–1645.

xxi As above.

xxii Cynthia Rousso, personal communication.

xxiii Chen, C., Hewitt, P.L. and Flett, G.L. (2015), 'Preoccupied Attachment, need to belong, shame and interpersonal perfectionism: An investigation of the Perfectionism Social Disconnection Model. Personality and Individual Differences'. *Personality and Individual Differences*, 76, 177–82.

xxiv Flett, G.L., Hewitt, P.L. Oliver, J.M. and McDonald, S. (2002), 'Perfectionism in Children and their Parents: A Developmental Analysis'. In G.L. Flett & L. Hewitt (Eds.) *Perfectionism: Theory, research, and treatment* (pp.89–132). Washington, DC: American Psychological Association

xxv Everett, G.E., Hupp, S.D.A. and Olmi, D.J. (2010), 'Time-out with Parents: A Descriptive Analysis of 30 Years of Research'. *Education and Treatment of Children*, 33, 2.

xxvi Van den akker, A.L., Hoffenaar, P. and Overbeek, G. (2022), 'Temper Tantrums in Toddlers and Preschoolers: Longtitudinal

Associations with Adjustment Problems'. *J Dev Behave Pediatr.*, 43(7), 409–17.

xxvii Lepper, M., Greene, D. and Nisbett, R. (1973), 'Undermining Children's Intrinsic Interest with Extrinsic Reward: A Test of the "Overjustification" Hypothesis'. *Journal of Personality and Social Psychology*, 28(1), 129–37.

xxviii Gray, P., Lancy, D.F. and Bjorklund, D.F. (2023), 'Decline in Independent Activity as a Cause of Decline in Children's Mental Wellbeing: Summary of the Evidence'. *Journal of Pediatrics* (Feb 2023).

xxix (1/3/24), 'British children face "shorter, unhappier lives" from obesity.' *The Times*, London.

xxx The concept of nutrition and intuition is not mine. It comes from a wonderful book called *If Not Dieting, Then What?* by Rick Kausman (2014), Vermillion Press. that everyone in the world should read. I would also recommend Laura Thomas's (2019) *Just Eat It*. Bluebird.

xxxi Fioravanti, G., Benucci, S., Ceragioli, G. and Casale, S. (2021), 'How the Exposure to Beauty Ideals on Social Networking Sites Influences Body Image'. *Adolescent Research Review*, 7, 419–58.

xxxii Jacques Peretti's 2013 TV show *The Men Who Made Us Thin* investigated this. Sadly no longer available on iPlayer, but, is summarised here https://wellcomecollection.org/works/fnyc9gxr

xxxiii Nelson, P., et al. (2018), 'Is childhood obesity a child protection concern?' Technical Report. Doncaster Council/ Sheffield Hallam University.

xxxiv Memon, A. N., Gowda, A.S., Rallabhandi, B., Bidika, E., Fayyaz, H., Salib, M. and Cancarevic, I. (2020), 'Have Our Attempts to Curb Obesity Done More Harm Than Good?' *Cureus*, 12(9): e10275. DOI 10.7759/cureus.10275

xxxv Porter, T. (2022), *You Don't Understand Me: A Young Woman's Guide to Life*. Bonnier.

xxxvi Flett, G.L. and Hewitt, P.L. (2022), *Perfectionism in Children and Adolescence*. APA Books.

xxxvii Thompson, A.L. Mendez, M.A., Borja, J.B., Adair, L.S., Zimmer, R. and Bentley, M.E. (2009), 'Development and Validation of the Infant Feeding Style Questionnaire'. *Appetite*, 53(2), 210–21.

xxxviii Wood, A.C., et al. (2020), 'Caregiver Influences on Eating Behaviors in Young Children: A Scientific Statement From the American Heart Association'. *J Am Heart Assoc*: e014520. DOI: 10.1161/JAHA.119.014520

REFERENCES

xxxix Cullinane, C. and Montacute, R. (2023), 'Tutoring – The New Landscape'. The Sutton Trust.

xl Parenting priorities: international attitudes towards raising children. The UK in the World Values Survey (2023). The Policy Institute at Kings College. https://www.worldvaluessurvey.org/WVSNewsShowMore.jsp?evYEAR=2023&evMONTH=-1

xli Dweck, C. (2012), *Mindset and How You Can Fill Your Potential.* Constable and Robinson.

xlii Ericsson, K.A. (2006), 'The Influence of Experience and Deliberate Practice on the Development of Superior Expert Performance'. Chapter 38 in Ericsson, K.A., Charness, N., Feltvich, P.J. and Hoffman, R.R. (Eds), *The Cambridge Handbook of Expertise and Expert Performance.* Cambridge University Press.

xliii Gladwell, M. (2008), *Outliers. The Story of Success.* Little, Brown and Company.

xliv Gary Lineker – 'Shut Up and Let Them Play': https://www.youtube.com/watch?v=EJ58O1izyJo

xlv Segalov, M. (30/4/2023), 'What if you don't make it?' *Guardian.*

xlvi Curran, T. and Hill, A.P. (2017), 'Perfectionism Is Increasing Over Time: A Meta-Analysis of Birth Cohort Differences From 1989 to 2016'. *Psychological Bulletin*, 145(4), 410–29.

xlvii Sahlberg, P. (2012), 'How GERM is infecting schools around the world'. Blog on Pasisahlberg.com

xlviii PA News agency report on the basis of a Freedom of Information request. Reported 3/1/23 in most quality national newspapers.

xlix Briefing by the Health Foundation (2022), 'Improving children and young people's mental health services'.

l 'Good Childhood Report' (2022). The Children's Society.

li World Health Organization (2020), 'Health Behaviour in School Aged Children'. https://gateway.euro.who.int/en/indicators/hbsc_44-pressured-by-schoolwork/visualizations/#id=27044

lii BBC *Today* programme (10/2/2017). Also at https://www.bbc.co.uk/news/education-38923034

liii Elliott, J.G., (2020) 'It's Time to Be Scientific About Dyslexia'. *Reading Research Quarterly*, 55(S1) pf S61–75.

liv NatCen(2019), 'How does poor mental health in the early years of secondary school impact on GCSE attainment?' Economic and Social Research Council.

lv Hodgkinson, T. (2009), *The Idle Parent.* Penguin.

REFERENCES

lvi   Flett, G.L. and Hewitt, P.L. (2022), *Perfectionism in Childhood and Adolescence: A Developmental Approach.* American Psychological Association.

lvii   https://www.statista.com/statistics/267963/participation-in-us-high-school-soccer

lviii   Haidt, J. (2024), *The Anxious Generation: How the Great Rewiring of Childhood is Causing an Epidemic of Mental Illness.* Penguin.

lix   Odgers, C. (4/4/2024), 'The great rewiring; unplugged'. *Nature*, 628.

lx   Odgers, C. and Jensen, M. (2020), 'Adolescent development and growing divides in the digital age'. *Dialogues in Clinical Neuroscience*, 22(2).

lxi   Przybylski, A. and Weinstein, K (2107), 'A Large-Scale Test of the Goldilocks Hypothesis: Quantifying the Relations Between Digital Screen Use and the Mental Well-Being of Adolescents'. Association for Psychological Science, 28(2), 204–15.

lxii   'Children's Media Lives (2024) Ten years of longtitudinal research'. A report for Ofcom.

lxiii   Kaiser Family Foundation Study (2010) Generation M^2 Media in the Lives of 8–18 year olds. https://www.kff.org/wp-content/uploads/2013/01/8010.pdf

lxiv   Adapted from Porter, T. (2024), *The You Don't Understand Me Journal.* Bonnier.

lxv   Haidt, J. (2024), *The Anxious Generation: How the Great Rewiring of Childhood is Causing an Epidemic of Mental Illness.* Penguin.

lxvi   Sigman, A. (2019), 'A Movement for Movement Screen time, physical activity and sleep: a new integrated approach for children'. https://www.api-play.org

lxvii   Vandenbosch, L., Fardouly, J. and Tiggemann, M. (2022), 'Social media and body image: Recent trends and future directions'. *Current Opinion in Psychology*, 45, 101289.

lxviii   Anderson, C.A., Shibuya, A., Ihori, N., Swing, E.L., Bushman, B.J., Sakamoto, A., Rothstein, H.R and Saleem, M. (2010), 'Violent Video Game Effects on Aggression, Empathy and Prosocial Behaviour in Eastern and Western Countries: A Meta-Analytic Review'. *Psychological Bulletin*, 136(2), 151–73.

lxix   Koolstra, C.M., van Zanten, J., Lucassen, N. and Ishaak, N. (2004), 'The formal pace of Sesame Street over 26 years, *Perceptual and Motor Skills*, 99(1), 354–60.

REFERENCES

lxx Beyens, I., Valkenburg, P.M. and Piotrowski, J.T. (2018), 'Screen media use and ADHD-related behaviors: Four decades of research'. *Proceedings of the National Academy of Sciences.* 115 (40), 9875–9881.

lxxi Haidt, J. (2024), *The Anxious Generation: How the Great Rewiring of Childhood is Causing an Epidemic of Mental Illness.* Penguin.

lxxii Fineberg, N.A., et al. (2022), 'Advances in problematic usage of the internet research – A narrative review by experts from the European network for problematic usage of the internet'. *Comprehensive Psychiatry*, 118, 152346.

lxxiii Fitzpatrick, C., et al. (2024), 'Early-Childhood Tablet Use and Outbursts of Anger'. *Jama Paediatrics.* doi:10.1001/jamapediatrics.2024.2511

lxxiv Yeager, D.S., Dahl, R.E. and Dweck, C.S. (2018), 'Why Interventions to Influence Adolescent Behaviour often Fail but Could Succeed'. *Perspect Psychol Sci*, 13(1); 1010–122.

lxxv Nagata, J., et al. (2024), 'Associations between media parenting practices and early adolescent screen use'. *Nature*, 5 June 2024

lxxvi André, F., et al. (2020) 'Gaming addiction, problematic gaming and engaged gaming – Prevalence and associated characteristics'. *Addictive Behaviors Report*, 12. 100324.

lxxvii Ofcom (2024), 'Children and Parents: Media Use and Attitudes Report'.

lxxviii Anderson, C.A., Shibuya, A., Ihori, N., Swing, E.L., Bushman, B.J., Sakamoto, A., Rothstein, H.R. and Saleem, M. (2010), 'Violent Video Game Effects on Aggression, Empathy and Prosocial Behaviour in Eastern and Western Countries: A Meta-Analytic Review'. *Psychological Bulletin*, 136(2), 151–73.

lxxix Niu, X., Li, J-Y., King, D.L., Rost, D.H., Wang, H-Z. and Wang, J-L. (2023), 'The relationship between parenting styles and adolescent problematic Internet use: A three-level meta-analysis'. *Journal of Behavioral Addictions.*

lxxx Children's Commissioner (Jan 2023), 'A lot of it actually is just abuse.' Young People and Pornography.

lxxxi Sommet, N. and Berent, J. (2022) Porn use and men's and women's sexual performance: evidence from a large longtitudinal sample. *Psychological Medicine*, 1-10.

lxxxii Children's Commissioner (Jan 2023), 'A lot of it actually is just abuse'. Young People and Pornography.

REFERENCES

lxxxiii Abrahamsson, S. (2024), 'Smartphone Bans, Student Outcome and Mental Health'. *Institutt for samfunnsøkonomi*. Department of Economics.

lxxxiv Travel to School. National Travel Survey 2014. Department for Transport.

lxxxv https://www.theguardian.com/uk-news/2023/aug/09/nearly-two-fifths-of-robberies-in-london-last-year-were-for-mobile-phones

lxxxvi Curran, T. and Hill, P. (2017), 'Perfectionism Is Increasing Over Time: A Meta-Analysis of Birth Cohort Differences From 1989 to 2016'. *Psychological Bulletin*, 145 (4), 410–29.

lxxxvii (12/11/24), 'Youth worklessness hits 10-year-high amid mental health crisis'. *The Times*.

lxxxviii Porter, T. (7 Feb 2024), 'The Lost Children of Education'. *Tes magazine*.

lxxxix Luthar, S.S., Kumar, N.L. and Zillmar, N. (2019), 'High-Achieving Schools Connote Risks for Adolescents: Problems Documented, Processes Implicated, and Directions for Intervention'. *American Psychologist*. Ibid.

xc As above.

xci (29/7/2024), 'Order! Gen Z's in the House – meet the twentysomething MPs.' *The Times*.

xcii Stiles, K., Lee, S.S. and Luthar, S.S. (2020), 'When Parents Seek Perfection: Implications for Psychological Functioning Among Teens at High-Achieving Schools'. *Journal of Child and Family Studies*, 29, 3117–128.

xciii Porter, T. (22 May 2022), 'Phones are like a scab we know we shouldn't pick: the truth about social media and anxiety'. *Guardian*.

xciv See the work of Marika Tiggemann https://www.flinders.edu.au/people/marika.tiggemann and Renee Engeln at http://bodyandmedia.com for a comprehensive exploration of these issues.

xcv Children's Commissioner (2023), 'A lot of it actually is just abuse': Young People and Pornography.

xcvi Smith, M. (7/9/2023), 'One in six boys aged 6–15 have a positive view of Andrew Tate'. YouGov.

xcvii Gladwell, M. (2008), *Outliers. The Story of Success*. Little, Brown and Company.

xcviii Iranzo-Tatay, C., Gimeno-Clemente, N., Barberá-Fons, M., Rodriguez-Campayo, M.A., Rojo-Bofill, L., Livianos-Aldana, L., Beato-Fernandez, L., Vaz-Leal, F. and Rojo-Moreno, L., 'Genetic and environmental

REFERENCES

contributions to perfectionism and its common factors'. *Psychiatry Research*. http://dx.doi.org/10.1016/j.psychres.2015.11.020.

xcix Flett, G. L. and Hewitt, P. L. (2022), 'Perfectionism in Childhood and Adolescence: A Developmental Approach'. American Psychological Association.

c Flett, G.L., Hewitt, P.L., Oliver, J.M. and Macdonald, S. (2002), 'Perfectionism in Children and Their Parents: A Developmental Analysis. In Perfectionism: Theory, Research and Treatment'. Ed. by G.L. Flett and P.L. Hewitt. American Psychological Association.

ci Curran, T. and Curran, H. (2022), 'Young People's Perceptions of Their Parents' Expectations and Criticism Are Increasing Over Time: Implications for Perfectionism'. *Psychological Bulletin*, 148(1-2), 107–28.

cii Luthar, S.S., Kumar, N.L. and Zillmar, N. (2019), 'High-Achieving Schools Connote Risks for Adolescents: Problems Documented, Processes Implicated, and Directions for Intervention'. *American Psychologist*.

ciii Fry, P.S. and Debats, D.L. (2009), 'Perfectionism and the five factor personality traits as predictors of mortality in older adults'. *Journal of Health Psychology* 14 (4) 513–24.

civ Curran, T. and Curran, H. (2022), 'Young People's Perceptions of Their Parents' Expectations and Criticism Are Increasing Over Time: Implications for Perfectionism'. *Psychological Bulletin*, 148(1-2), 107–28.

cv Yeager, D.S., Dahl, R.E., and Dweck, C.S. (2018), 'Why Interventions to Influence Adolescent Behaviour often Fail but Could Succeed'. *Perspect Psychol Sci*, 13(1); 1010–122.

cvi Weinstein, N., Legate, N., Ryan, W.S. and Hemmy, L. (2018), 'Autonomous orientation predicts longevity: New findings from the Nun study'. *Journal of Personality*, 87, 181–93.

cvii See Nancy Darling (28/3/11), 'Why Do Teens Lie? Part 1'. *Psychology Today*.

INDEX

ability, innate 125–6, 127, 144, 226
abuse 20, 24, 109, 164, 199
academic pressure 144, 145, 147–53, 213, 215–22, 239, 249
activities 124, 128–31, 133, 160, 239
addiction 187, 193, 197
ADHD 102–3, 148, 149, 152, 169, 187
adolescence 147–8, 180, 196, 207–81
advice, unsolicited 266–7, 279
aggression 169, 170, 198, 224, 225
Ainsworth, Mary 31
anger 212, 257
anorexia 112, 237, 249, 272
anxiety 6–7, 26–9, 101, 102, 147, 169, 212, 219, 224, 266
  parental 136, 240, 277–8
  and perfectionism 69, 70, 143, 227, 228
apologising 270–2, 276
appearance-driven culture 107–8, 224
assessments, educational 149–50, 152
attachment 22, 30–41, 44, 56, 58, 93, 120, 158–9, 161, 166, 193–4
attention 161, 194–7
autonomy 10, 239, 245, 252–3, 269

babies 15–70, 73
backing down 82–3, 245
balance 62, 64, 115–16, 117, 118, 153, 163–4, 270
bedtimes 161–2, 178
behaviour theory and management 43–53, 74, 75, 83, 85, 86–91, 187–97
body image, social media and 107–8, 224
bonds see attachment
boredom 187, 195

boundaries: babies 63
  in adolescence 230, 232, 241–7, 250, 264, 272, 280
  in childhood 188, 189–90, 198, 203
  toddlers and 83, 115, 116, 118–19
Bowlby, John 31
Brown, Brené 25, 164
burnout 147, 227, 228
busyness 123–34, 135, 153, 159, 160, 162, 195, 211, 214, 222

CAMHS 103, 169
Carling, Sam 221
central-heating parenting 259–60, 264, 272, 281
child-led play 95–9, 104, 158, 159–60, 163, 165
childcare 58–60, 61
childhood 121–206
Children's Society, Good Childhood survey 148
chores 99, 239, 259
Chua, Amy, *Battle Hymn of the Tiger Mother* 126
cold parenting 75, 76
communication 95, 97, 159, 160, 167, 204
comparison 66, 67, 103, 132, 211, 214, 219, 222, 223–4, 229
compassion 152, 270
competence, emotional 9, 58, 69, 84–5, 147, 176, 205, 232, 233, 234, 272, 278–9
competition 211, 217, 219, 221
compliance 82, 91, 98, 99, 131, 190–4, 196, 230, 242, 243, 246, 247–9, 259, 260

INDEX

compromise 276, 280
confidence 128, 191
connections 159, 194–7, 205
consequences 44, 79, 82, 86, 90, 92, 98, 192, 196, 198
consistency 80–2, 123–4, 155, 237–8
containment 189, 241
control 101, 227
criticism 221–2, 227, 267, 279
crying, controlled 45, 51
curiosity 85, 172–7, 230, 264, 268

dependence, breeding 144, 249
depression 8, 52, 70, 101, 169, 219, 228
diagnoses 6, 150–2
dieting 108, 113, 118
disconnection 111, 187
dissatisfaction 102, 108, 187, 224, 225
downtime 129, 145, 187
drugs 7, 197, 266, 272
Dweck, Carol 125
dyslexia 148, 149, 151–2

eating and food 105–20, 276
  eating disorders 70, 102, 105, 110–12, 147, 212, 224
education 135–56, 211, 215–22, 225, 229
emotions 54, 176
  emotional competence 9, 58, 84–5, 69, 147, 176, 205, 232, 233, 234, 272, 278–9
empathy 85, 101, 158, 172–7, 198, 230, 247, 264, 268
Erikson, Erik 213–14
expectations 24, 27, 38, 66–8, 70, 126–7, 129–30, 132, 144, 201, 211, 212, 221–2, 229, 249
externalisation 168–9
extreme parenting 86–91, 128, 141, 150, 165

Federer, Roger 240
feelings 6–7, 260–1
  naming and acknowledging 9, 83, 90, 91, 176
firm parenting 75, 76, 230, 250, 264, 272–3

firm and kind parenting 42–53, 75, 76, 117, 178, 181–5, 195, 196, 198, 202, 205
  sledgehammer firm 193, 200, 201, 202, 205
food and eating 105–20, 276
football 126–7, 168, 231
Ford, Gina 25, 46–7, 63, 75
free play 99–104, 129, 147, 160
Freud, Lucien 43
friends 235, 237, 239, 265, 279
  on/off friends 166–7, 223
  relationships in childhood 157, 158, 164–77
fun 91, 162–4
the future, looking towards 61–2, 146

gaming 179, 181–2, 187, 197–8, 203, 211, 224
Gates, Bill 128
Gawdat, Mo 24
GCSEs 215–16
gender 32
  play and 167–9
gentle parenting 83–91, 188
Gladwell, Malcolm, *Outliers* 125–6, 128, 131
Global Education Reform Movement (GERM) 138, 139, 145, 215
'good girls' 247–9, 253, 257, 260, 267
Gray, Peter 101
growth mindset 125, 218

Haidt, Jonathan, *The Anxious Generation* 186
happiness and joy 7–8, 24, 146, 155, 162, 277
hard work 124–6, 127, 128, 134, 144, 156, 214, 220
Harlow, Harry 31–2
helicopter parents 213
holding on 234–53
hunger 105, 113, 116, 117, 120

ideas, sharing 100
identity 224–5, 234, 237, 243, 247
  identity crisis 213–14
  as a parent 54–70, 177

INDEX

imperfection 27–8, 231, 271, 276
independence 9–10, 73–4, 144, 170, 175, 195, 196, 230, 232, 234, 241, 279
individualism 112, 125
influence 211, 256–60
interactions 37, 75
internalisation 168–9
the internet 66–8, 70, 132, 178–206, 211, 214, 222–5
intervention 171–2, 272–3, 274
intuition 106, 112, 116, 117, 119
IQ 149, 151

joy 7–8, 146, 162, 277
Jung, Carl 28

Karmel, Annabel 112
Kausman, Rick, *If Not Dieting, Then What?* 106
kind parenting 75, 76
Kipling, Rudyard 276
Klein, Melanie 43

Lagarde, Christine 62
lax parenting 75, 76, 195
learned helplessness 52, 212
learning, play and 92, 96–7, 101
letting go 234–53, 260–4
Lineker, Gary 126–7, 143, 231
listening, active 264–70
Lorenz, Konrad 32
love, unconditional 145, 159
lying 263

marginal gains parenting 60
May, Katherine, *The Electricity of Every Living Thing* 35–6
Men Are from Mars, Women Are from Venus 267
mental health 13, 42, 101, 174–5, 182
  academic pressure 135, 137, 147–53, 154, 218, 221–2
  adolescents and 209–13, 216, 226–7, 272
  good mental health 5–10, 12–13, 270
mindset 73–4
  growth mindset 125, 218
money 257–9, 262

National Curriculum 138–9
NHS Child and Adolescent Mental Health Services in England 148
nursery school 60, 61
nutrition 106, 112, 116, 117, 119

Obama, Michelle 130
obesity 105, 109, 110–11, 112
Online Safety Act (2023) 179
outcome-based parenting 136, 183, 188, 248
overeating 107, 109, 110–12

parents: of adolescent and adult children 275–81
parent-pause listening 266–7
parenting-as-a-verb concept 21–2, 126
peak parenting 21, 23, 69–70, 126
play and 92, 93–104
your identity as a parent 54–70
partial reinforcement schedule 45, 82
Pavlov, Ivan 43–4, 89, 190, 191
people pleasers 191, 263
perfectionism 18–19, 22, 23, 24, 86–91, 103, 111, 132, 166, 248–9
  academic 142–3, 156, 249
  feeding your child and 119–20
  and identity 65–70
  and mental health 212, 221–2, 227, 228
  perfect parenting standards 225–33
phones 132, 178–206, 209, 213, 214, 276
physical punishment 74–5, 82
play 91, 92–104, 187
  child-led play 95–9, 104, 158, 159–60, 163, 165
  commodification of 96, 101, 102
  free play 99–104, 129, 147, 160
  gender and 167–9
  and learning opportunities 92, 96–7, 101
porn 179, 198, 199–201, 224, 225, 266
praise 78, 188, 191, 229, 248
pre-schoolers and toddlers 71–120
present moment, living in the 146
pressure 212
  academic 144, 145, 147–53, 213, 215–22, 239, 249
problems, solving 267–9
Przybylski, Andrew 181–2

INDEX

punishments 74–5, 82, 188, 192, 193, 257
  time out 75, 76, 79–83, 85, 91

qualifications 135, 139, 141, 144, 150, 152, 153, 211, 215–16, 217

reading 124, 143, 145, 149, 151, 161
rebellion 191, 238, 243–7, 248, 257
reciprocity 9, 94–5, 98, 100, 117, 165, 232
relationships 8–9
  in childhood 157–77, 188
  keeping relationships going 158–62, 254–74
  relationship-based parenting 30–41, 52, 55, 92, 93–104, 145
resentment 68–9
resilience 8, 147, 213, 239
restraint 115, 116
restrictive eating 110–12
Robinson, Ken 219–20
Rousso, Cynthia 65
routines 46–7, 63, 123–4, 155, 162, 189–90, 193
rudeness 257, 259, 263
rules 189–90, 193, 239, 250, 256
rupture and repair 37–40, 158

Sahlberg, Paul 138
Samuel, Julia 54, 128
SATS 139, 154, 155
scaffolding 100, 101, 164–5, 194–7, 232, 252
school and education 21, 109, 123–4, 126, 131, 132, 135–56, 201–2, 211, 215–22, 225, 229
screens 132, 178–206, 209, 214
self-esteem 8, 129–30, 152, 153, 228, 277
self-harm 8, 129, 143, 147, 212, 228, 247, 249, 260–1, 266
self-improvement 22, 125, 131, 132, 143, 211, 212, 214, 228, 230, 239
separation 10, 31, 234–53, 254–5, 269, 277
sexual content 179, 198, 199–201, 224, 225, 266
Shakespeare, William 256
sharing 100
Skinner, B. F. 43
sleep 42–53, 161–2

social media 66–8, 70, 107–8, 175, 180, 181–2, 213, 222–5
standards 25–6, 66, 132, 215, 225–33
star charts 75, 76, 78, 88–9, 127, 248
Still Face Experiment 36–7, 93, 120
success 126–8, 214, 229, 231
  academic 140, 141–3, 144–7, 219–20
Supernanny 75, 76
Sure Start 77, 95–6
Swift, Taylor 130, 248
synchronicity 120, 165, 232

tantrums 79–91
Tate, Andrew 224
teenagers and tweens 67, 89, 131, 207–81
theory of mind 100, 167–8
Thompson, A. L. 117
Thorndike, Edward 43
Tiger Mums 63, 64
time out 75, 76, 79–83, 85, 91
tipping points 118, 128–31, 181–2
toddlers and pre-schoolers 60, 71–120
Tronick, Dr Ed 36–7
Tutu, Desmond 5
tweens and teens 67, 89, 131, 207–81
twenty-four-hour-contact style parenting 38–40

uber-relaxed parents 63, 64
unhappiness 123, 148, 218
university 220–1, 222

validation 129–30, 252
values 134, 183–5, 202, 203, 205
vulnerability 25, 65, 96, 270, 271

watching 264–70
Watson, John B. 43
Webster-Stratton Incredible Years 95–6
WhatsApp 223
Wilkinson, Jonny 23, 25, 145
Winnicott, Donald 19, 27–8
work, parental life and 56–62
World Health Organization (WHO) 148

Youth Offending Teams 169